Survival Retreats

A Prepper's Guide to Creating a Sustainable, Defendable Refuge

David Black

Foreword by James C. Jones

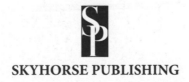

SKYHORSE PUBLISHING

Cover: An artist's rendition of an effective retreat, with high ground, difficult remote terrain, and a structure designed to provide cover and firepower from multiple directions and on all sides.

Skyhorse Publishing books may be purchased in bulk at special discounts for sales promotion, corporate gifts, fund-raising, or educational purposes. Special editions can also be created to specifications. For details, contact the Special Sales Department, Skyhorse Publishing, 307 West 36th Street, 11th Floor, New York, NY 10018 or info@skyhorsepublishing.com.

Skyhorse® and Skyhorse Publishing® are registered trademarks of Skyhorse Publishing, Inc. ®, a Delaware corporation.

www.skyhorsepublishing.com

10 9 8 7 6 5 4 3 2 1

Library of Congress Cataloging-in-Publication Data is available on file.

Print ISBN: 978-1-5107-2540-9
Ebook ISBN: 978-1-5107-2541-6

Printed in the United States of America

Survival Retreats

Contents

Foreword by
James C. Jones

THE SUBJECT OF SURVIVAL RETREATS, BUNKERS, AND SHELTERS OF various types has been addressed in numerous fiction and nonfiction books since the beginning of the Cold War. Throughout the latter half of the twentieth century, the focus of the subject was primarily directed at sheltering from the blast effects and radioactive fallout that would result from the detonation of nuclear weapons. The twenty-first century brought with it a broader variety of threat scenarios that could require various kinds of shelters and retreats. Today's would-be survivor must prepare for a matrix of interrelated threats and multiple disaster situations that may require sheltering in place or evacuation to a near or remote location. While the need for a Cold War bomb shelter or fallout shelter was seen as a precaution against an event that might happen, today's imperatives for shelter and retreat concepts are necessitated by worsening and multiplying perils that are happening and cannot be ignored.

Every news cycle brings revelations of new storms, droughts, wildfires, crime waves, civil disorder, international tensions, and economic instability. The security of our homes and communities becomes more and more fragile and the necessity of having a safe place to go grows more imperative each year. Having the capability to isolate oneself and the ones we care for from epidemics, lawlessness, chaos, and other hazards while providing all of the necessities for life, safety, and health is the most important mission that any responsible citizen of today's world can undertake. The decision of if and when to flee to a preplanned retreat or to shelter in place is one of the most difficult and important choices that must be made during a truly massive and long-lasting disaster, but such a decision can only be made if the survivor has preplanned and established facilities for these options well in advance.

This book goes beyond simply providing the physical specifications and requirements of shelter building and retreat establishment. The equally important subjects of decision-making, budgeting, and realistic planning are addressed throughout. The first chapter, An Introduction to Survivalism, explores the philosophical foundations of survival thinking and the justification for preparedness. A section on the history of survival retreats through the ages reviews both successful and failed examples of various kinds of retreats from the Jews at Masada to the hardened bunkers of the Cold War era. The chapter on retreat strategies and management includes essential recommendations on how to select the right kind of retreat for the right kind of situation in the right location. Storage and stocking requirements for life-essential needs—including water, food, medical supplies, and weapons—is detailed. The importance of and techniques for networking with others to build your survival community is also outlined.

The physical aspects of establishing a retreat are covered in detail in chapter four. An examination of the critical relationship of the purpose of the shelter to its location and requirements is followed by well-organized and detailed descriptions of multiple types of retreats and shelters. The exigencies of remote and isolated "bug out" retreats and urban shelter-in-place or "bug in" retreats are equally well detailed. The prerequisites for the location of a remote retreat site as well as the choice of an in-home safe room or shelter are well defined. The inclusion of well-selected photographs of shelters, bunkers, supplies, and equipment adds interest and clarification to each subject. Actual construction instructions, supply sources, and design recommendations provide the reader with everything necessary to build the retreat or shelter that matches their needs. Great attention is given to shelter and home security measures and devices, including locks, alarms, surveillance cameras, and reinforcements of existing structures. Providing adequate electrical power utilizing solar panels is covered as an important aspect of extended survivability. Essential information on providing alternative emergency communications using CB, GMRS, and FRS radio walkie-talkies is included.

What you need and how much of each necessity is the focus of the food sustainability and supplementation chapter. In addition to the basic lists of supplies and equipment, there are specific recommendations with references to sources and websites. This section goes beyond just stocking up to cover sustainable methods of water gathering, food production, and recovery concepts. The reader will also find a step-by-step table establishing each survival retreat requirement focus, and the needed supplies and budget costs based on visits to actual functioning retreats will be of great aid to the reader.

There is no doubt that having a safe and sustainable retreat or urban shelter is going to necessitate passive and active defensive methods and weapons. Basic fortification, tactics, and weapons application is therefore thoroughly explored.

The aspects of establishing immediate and improvised retreats while travelling is covered in the final chapter. This important aspect of retreat establishment is often overlooked. This chapter is based on practical experiences in national and international travel. Being away from home and fare from access to any prepared retreat or shelter possess a daunting and unique set of requirements for establishing a secure retreat on the fly. Terrorist targeting of tourist areas and the increasing unpredictability of weather related disasters and even local unrest and crime make being able to establish security and survivability in hotels and on the road as important as having a remote retreat or a safe-room at home. Various methods, devices and precautions are related to this aspect of sheltering are detailed.

Whether you are a "hard core" survivalist preparing for a major, long-term cataclysm or a prepper just seeking to improve your security and expand your options for surviving natural or manmade disasters at home or away from home, you will find plenty of useful information and realistic advice in this book.

James C. Jones is the cofounder of Live Free USA, a national survival club and self-reliance organization. A certified hazard control manager and EMT, he has developed and conducted hundreds of survival training events and seminars over the past forty years and has written hundreds of articles for Live Free's newsletter, American Survivor. *He currently writes articles for several national preparedness and survival publications while continuing to teach a variety of survival courses and to make presentations at major preparedness expositions. His books include* Beyond Survival: An Introduction to the Self-Reliance Revolution *and* The Live Free Book of Total Survival.

Preface

THIS IS THE THIRD BOOK IN A TRILOGY OF WHAT COULD LOOSELY BE called a "survival" series. Twenty years ago, I wouldn't have ever imagined myself writing a series like this. I would not consider myself a survivalist in the current sense of the word. If I had to describe myself best, I think that the word "prepper" would be most appropriate, though probably not entirely accurate. It sounds wishy-washy, and that's most likely because I'm a moderate. I believe in *moderation,* and survivalism in the minds of most people is not considered moderate.

This book touches on everything—from construction, to power production and farming, to armed combat. In a volume this size, it would be impossible to provide a detailed discussion of everything that one could possibly want to know and understand about survival retreats. I just scratch the surface here. What you see is the tip of an enormous iceberg of knowledge.

In today's world, it only makes sense to be interactive with the most powerful source of public information available: the Internet, and it's right at our fingertips. This book refers to numerous websites where you, the reader, can find more detailed information than I am able to provide in this book. I highly recommend that you sit next to your computer or have your laptop handy while reading. Become one with your browser. Print off as much as you can afford, because if you truly do believe that the shit will someday hit the fan, then you believe the Internet will then be vulnerable and you will lose that resource when the service providers and servers crash.

Finally, as I have seen in my research, and as the world has witnessed so many times throughout history, survivalism and retreatism can be risky. Don't go off the deep end—it's bound to go bad. Just remember:

The world is not your enemy.
The zombie hordes have not been unleashed.
The world and civilization will still be here in 2013.
I promise

—DB

Chapter 1

Introduction to Survivalism

DEFINITION OF SURVIVALISM

So what is the difference between a prepper and a survivalist? Years from now, the definitions will still be obscure, but today there's an identifiable difference. For our purposes, let's define preppers as individuals or groups who actively prepare for minor-to-moderate disruptions in public works and services due to disasters or national emergencies that *might* be accompanied by brief glitches in political and social order. In other words, preppers do basic disaster preparation and planning, which may or may not include an emphasis on continuing self-sufficiency and sustainability (growing food and producing energy). This is a rational and reasonable idea, fueled by the understanding that we are not invulnerable to small- or large-scale disasters that could temporarily set us back in our standard of living and societal stability.

Preppers are often known to distrust politicians and the economy, but they usually have a basic belief in the continuity of community ethics and the survival of technology. They know that even if 90 percent of the world's population were snuffed out by a megapandemic, there would still be 30 million survivors in the United States alone. That's 700 million worldwide!

The survivors of this megapandemic would most likely include politicians, doctors, law officers, lawyers, firefighters, scientists, teachers, and technicians—the same cross section of the working world that existed before the event. The infrastructure might be temporarily shut down, but it would still remain structurally intact, as would the knowledge to build, repair, maintain, and manufacture. Our sheer numbers and the redundant storage of knowledge—from the brain pool and books to computer files and the Internet—ensures the eventual survival and revival of both society and technology once outbreaks of unrest and violence are addressed.

Survivalism, on the other hand, is a movement of individuals or groups who actively prepare for apocalyptic, cataclysmic disasters—natural or man-made—that result in societal and economic collapse and the breakdown of normal community protection systems, culminating in widespread pandemonium and chaos. This is "Prep-ism Gone Wild"—disaster planning with the added components of aggressive self-defense and fundamental survival measures to counter the resulting anarchy and lawless bedlam.

This book is on survival retreats, which can be defined as refuges for survivalists, and which are also known in survivalist terms as BOLs, or bug-out locations. Retreats run the gamut from a simple food storage cache at an individual's home apartment to massive fortified high-tech retreat communities. Retreats are generally intended to be well stocked, self-sufficient to varying degrees, sparse but comfortable, and easily defended. They are also usually located in low-populated rural areas.

The triad that characterizes survivalism consists of disaster preparation, self-defense, and wilderness survival. Unfortunately, survivalism often has overtones of violent political activism, conspiracy theorism, religious fanaticism, science fiction, and new age extremism—a world fraught with end-times apocalypse, Planet X, zombie attacks at dawn, alien invaders, and Soylent

Green. This vision of survivalism frightens most of us, as does the frequency with which survivalists are blamed for domestic terrorism and deadly conflicts with the government and law enforcement.

PSYCHOLOGY AND SOCIOLOGY OF SURVIVALISM AND SURVIVALIST RETREATS

American survivalists prior to 9/11 and Hurricane Katrina were most often males who had antigovernment sentiments and who were essentially preparing and waiting, perhaps hoping, for the final conflict. This group mainly consisted of individuals and groups who were ready to provide their own versions of civil defense and vigilante law, and the rest of us wondered if they were indeed far too dangerous to tolerate.

Except for some bad press caused by the occasional antigovernment or religious conflict, preppers and many survivalists went unrecognized, fitting into the crowd. Survialists, though, as opposed to preppers, seemed to be driven by darker plans, searching for trouble because trouble was one of the few places in society they seemed to fit in. In the movies, ordinary people become extraordinary heroes: Survivalists save the world and fix what's broken. It would be reasonable to assume that the opportunity to become indispensable was one of the big reasons many people were drawn to survivalism, a phenomenon discussed by Dr. Richard Mitchell in his book *Dancing at Armageddon*.

Closely examined, the popular interest in survivalism appears to be a reaction to certain influences, rather than being the result of a deliberate and orchestrated movement. Its popularity rises when current events are tragic or tense, and falls when threats are perceived to be absent. The lull in interest right after the end of the Cold War is a perfect example. Survivalism loses credibility when things seem right. On the other end of that scale, though, survivalism's popularity spikes when there's bad news; and with the economic crisis, credit crunch, environmental disasters, terrorism, war, pandemics, oil prices, and international saber rattling that has occurred since the 2000s, world events now appear to be giving survivalism some degree of credibility, and its popularity is enormous at the time of this writing. Many preppers, who for a long time were likely to be moderate liberals, are now feeling uneasy and are sliding to the right. The constant 24-7 bombardment of bad news by our modern communication technologies (Internet, cable news, satellite, etc.) and Hollywood media (*Cloverfield, I Am Legend, 28 Days of Night, Dawn of the Dead*) only fuels the nervousness of an already-worried population. Even so, survivalists are still eyed with a degree of mistrust—like a quiet, skulking dog that can't be trusted. This is in large part due to the common belief that retreats can only be effective if they are clandestine, as the public does not trust what they see as hidden or mysterious.

The purpose of this book is to help the average reader see survival retreats through more practical eyes—a rational practical step beyond basic disaster preparation. Religion, politics, and doomsday predictions will be absent from this text. Instead, the simple belief in the basic ethics and morality of modern Western society will be assumed.

Chapter 2

The History of the Survival Retreat

ANCIENT AND PRE-HISTORY

IF WE USE THE BASIC RETREAT CRITERIA GIVEN IN CHAPTER 1 (DEFENSIBLE, sustainable, and nonurban), then there's an unlimited amount of material to sift through. From Noah's ark, to the castles of Europe, to the Anasazi cliff dwellings, retreats have been a basic means of defense from impending threats. Much of the current understanding of tactical defense of retreats comes from ancient manuscripts and archaeology. A lot of it supports the concepts of modern survivalism. Some of it, on the other hand, does not. Look at the rebel Jewish fortress of Masada. Like several modern examples, the siege of Masada by the Romans ended in the murder-suicide of its residents—an example of how political activism and religious extremism in the atmosphere of survivalism can combine with tragic results.

RECENT HISTORY

Many of the books we read and movies we watch are based on survival stories, and many of these contain elements of survival retreats. One interesting fact-based example is the story of the Bielski brothers in Belarus during World War II. You can rent the movie *Defiance* (2008) for this historical yet Hollywood version of a successful Red Dawn–style retreat. *The Diary of Anne Frank*, which is one of the most famous stories of the 20th century, was set in Nazi-occupied Holland during World War II. The retreat that she and her family used was successful for an extended period of time, but ultimately did not last.

The atrocities of World War II highlight some interesting points about survivalists and survivalism. One crucial point of

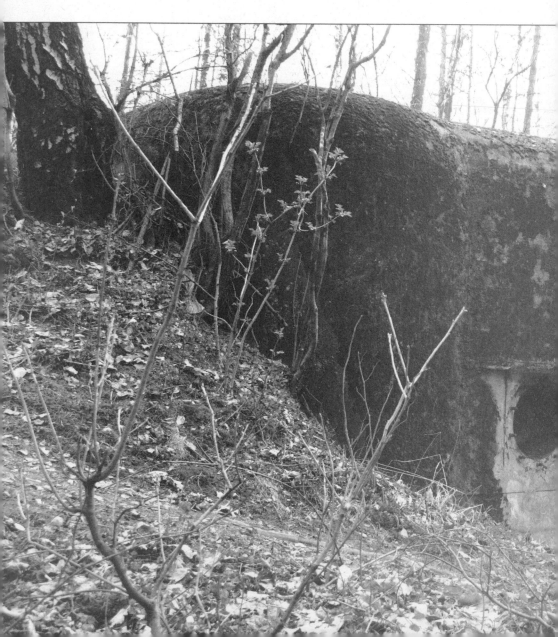

survivalism is that it doesn't work unless there's a clear "trip wire" (as Ragnar Benson, a prolific survivalist writer, puts it). Exactly what will it take for the survivalist to go into retreat mode? History has shown that denial and stalling to "finish up a few things" before leaving for safety or fighting back can lead to a deadly complacency.

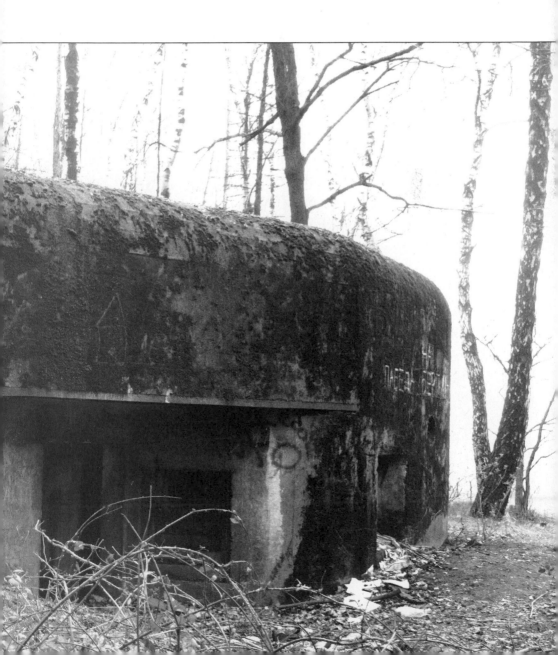

Another good read is the tale of the Utah War, an 1857 invasion by federal forces against the Mormons' western retreat in the Salt Lake Valley. You can look it up on the Internet for various versions of the story. That community retreat was established in an attempt to escape the hostility of federal and local governments. In the end, the federal troops prevailed, but the remoteness of the retreat and the defense strategy of the Mormon militia successfully delayed the invasion and averted the extermination of the Mormon community.

MODERN HISTORY
The Cold War Era

This is the period of time that begins in 1949 and goes on until the breakup of the Soviet Union in 1991. Fallout shelters, the precursors of modern family and community retreats, were first considered in 1949 when President Truman announced that the Soviet Union had the atomic bomb. The Gaither Report, a 1957 assessment of the nuclear capabilities and civil defense of the two nuclear powers, increased this interest. In 1958, the Office of Civil Defense began promoting the idea of home bomb shelters and provided several how-to manuals on how to build, supply, and prepare them.

Three incidents occurred during the Kennedy years that stunned and terrified the public, cementing our insecurities about the threat of nuclear war and our ability to defend our shores:

1. The Berlin Wall Crisis
2. The Cuban Missile Crisis
3. The assassination of President Kennedy

These events, and a handful of other dreadful incidents—such as the North Korean attack and confiscation of the *USS Pueblo* and the napalm bombing of the *USS Liberty* by our supposed ally, Israel—marked a turning point in popular thinking about disaster preparedness for the United States. The general public was now thinking about not just the threat of nuclear war, but also of inflation, supply shortages, infrastructure failures, and governmental collapse. Kennedy launched an effort to install bomb and fallout shelters across the United States after the events of the Cuban Missile Crisis. In 1967, the team of architect Don Stephens and investment analyst Harry Browne began giving seminars on surviving an economic collapse and how to build and equip survival retreats in select remote locations. Subsequently, there appeared a number of books and articles on personal preparedness written by Stephens and other writers including Howard Ruff, Mel Tappan, and Kurt Saxon.

After the return of the crew of the *USS Pueblo* from North Korean imprisonment, and as America began to focus on the mess overseas in Vietnam, domestic defense began to seem unimportant, and interest in shelters fell. Many were converted to storage rooms, wine cellars, or recreation rooms.

In spite of the apparent disinterest in the 1970s, a number of books by popular authors advocated moving to rural areas and building fortified, well-equipped retreats to defend against plundering. The terms "retreat" and "retreater" were often used to describe the location and the individual. Later on, "survivalist" became the preferred term to describe the retreater culture.

A further decline in interest in survivalism came after the United States pulled out of Vietnam in 1973, which briefly left us with the perception that we were less threatening to or threatened by the Soviet Union and China. But the disturbing truth was that we had lost a war to a tiny, third-world nation, and that realization eventually brought upon a surge of Cold War paranoia in the late 70s and early 80s. It probably was fostered even more by the economic collapse of Mexico and the American involvement in

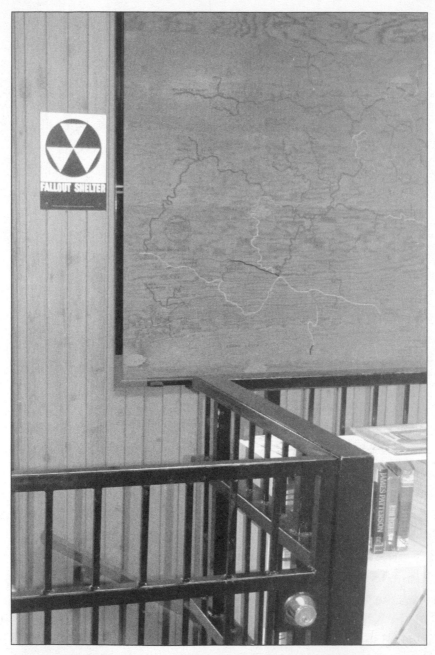

Many of the 1960s' fallout shelters still remain intact with the antiquated survival supplies covered in dust. This one is located in the basement of a small-town library in the Southwest.

potentially disastrous conflicts in Central America and Africa. In addition, conservative Americans watched in I-told-you-so fashion as the Soviet Union invaded Afghanistan and young anticommunist insurgents waged a successful war against the intruders.

It was during this period of increased paranoia over Cuban and Soviet influence in those regions that Hollywood released two very influential survivalist movies: *First Blood* (1982), the story of Rambo, and *Red Dawn* (1984), an ultimate piece of survivalism propaganda. The premise for *Red Dawn* was of a group of small-town high school football jocks who become insurgent heroes in the fight against the communist invasion of Mid-America. Gun laws were slammed in a scene in which the Soviet and Cuban armies used Firearms Transaction Records (Form 4473) to track down local gun owners. The bumper-sticker ditty "They can have my gun when they pry it from my cold dead hand" was ushered into scripture status when the film showed a Cuban soldier prying a gun from the hands of a dead patriot. *Red Dawn* couldn't help but appeal directly to every right-wing male. The concept of the invading horde screwing with the holy trinity— guns, alcohol, and football—evoked daydreams of heroism in every conservative, man and boy. The film, which was remade in 2010, stands as the single-most influential piece of survivalist proselytism in the media today.

At about the same time (1985), the TV series *MacGyver* began its seven-year, 139-episode run. The character MacGyver was distinctly liberal and antigun (he used a gun only once in the entire series), and some twenty episodes had antagonist survival-ist or retreat subthemes. But MacGyver was handy with anything, from duct tape to a knife. Survivalists fell in love with his ability to improvise a happy ending in the face of catastrophe and against all odds. He is religiously touted today on many survivalist websites as the quintessential survivalist, and among survivalists the question "What would Jesus do?" has been replaced by "What would MacGyver do?" Almost twenty-five years later, *Burn Notice* took over where *MacGyver* left off, giving hard-core survivalists a modern high-tech fed-shafted urban retreater to idolize, one who's not afraid to take a few feds down wherever he goes.

Interest in survivalism tanked again after the dissolution of the Soviet Union in 1991. Red Dawners were sorely disillusioned. But a series of events in the American West would soon make them feel at home again.

The New Millennium

Randy Weaver's retreat at Ruby Ridge is the classic example of a modern retreat gone awry. Weaver was a blue-collar, ex–Green Beret worker from Iowa, before he moved his family to Northern Idaho in 1983. The purpose of this move was to escape what the family considered to be a "corrupt society." His wife was a religious woman who believed the apocalypse was just around the corner and the family should prepare to survive the impending doom in the wilderness. Some unfortunate dealings with firearms and associations with local activists attracted the attention of law enforcement, ATF, and the FBI. These dealings eventually led to criminal charges against Mr. Weaver. Misunderstandings on both sides led to several nonlethal conflicts that prompted the authorities to place his property and movements under close surveillance. By 1992, federal law enforcement personnel began to see ex–Green Beret Weaver and his retreat as a serious threat, and the fears were fueled by reports of a dangerous cache of weapons and a system of booby traps and tunnels at the retreat, as well as rumors that Weaver had threatened to shoot anyone trying to arrest him.

What resulted was a violent confrontation that left Weaver's wife and fourteen-year-old son killed. His son had been shot in the back by a federal officer when he reacted to an alert by the family dog. His wife was shot by a federal sniper as she stood in the cabin doorway holding their ten-month-old baby. This incident brought enormous attention and some sympathy to the survivalist movement. The general public was outraged, and when the scenario was replayed in even more horrific fashion at a religious retreat in Waco, Texas, a year later, survivalism became the Robin Hood of American conservatism. Timothy McVeigh, who was the mastermind of the Oklahoma City bombing in 1995, considered the worst single act of domestic terrorism in United States history, stated that the Ruby Ridge and Waco murders were the motivation for his actions.

Probably the most classic read on hard-core retreating is Ragnar Benson's 1998 booklet, *The Modern Survival Retreat*. It's packed with tons of truly good practical information and ideas, as well as revealing insights into retreater psychology. It's very well written and easy to read and understand by beginners and professionals alike. Interestingly enough, this book seems to be a lesson in paranoia and appears to be more of a reaction to federal aggression at the Ruby Ridge and Waco tragedies than a focused look at more reasonable preparations for massive disasters or the long-term meltdown of society. Benson defines retreaters as individuals or groups who go into "voluntary, domestic seclusion." He postulates that the first key to successful retreating is to identify who the enemy is, and Benson thus gives us an insight into the real difference between preppers and survivalists. Preppers prepare for events, while survivalists prepare for enemies. The enemy in Benson's book is not the zombie horde or foreign invaders, the enemy is definitively the federal government.

These events and the resulting media coverage made everyone very nervous, and a lot of attention—much of it negative—was focused on the survivalism movement. After Oklahoma City, the term "survivalist" took on an aura of insane fanaticism, but Y2K loomed in the near future. As the time came closer, the predictions of technological chaos and pandemonium grew by leaps and bounds, and the demand for prepper and survivalist knowledge and skills grew with it.

In spite of the fact that the anticipated technological Armageddon of Y2K didn't happen, the boom of interest in survivalism and retreats continued, and in the vernacular of the survivalism industry, the shit hit the fan in America and throughout the whole world:

- September 11, 2001: Islamic terrorists hijack four U.S. airliners and crash them into the Pentagon and the World Trade Center, causing nearly 3,000 deaths.
- September 18, 2001: Anthrax attacks are launched by mail against media and government targets.
- October 7, 2001: America goes to war in response to the tragedy of September 11. The United States and United Kingdom commence the first attack on the Taliban and Al-Qaeda in Afghanistan.
- November 26, 2001: The United States officially admits a recession is in progress. The rising unemployment rate and a failing stock market had been headlines in the news for months. The collapse of the dot-coms and the 9/11 attacks compounded the economic situation, and various accounting scandals started to run rampant.
- November 25, 2002: Security-related federal agencies are consolidated and reorganized, and from that, the Department of Homeland Security is born. The DHS and FEMA launch campaigns to encourage individual preparation for such ugly threats as biological, chemical, and nuclear terrorism.
- March 19, 2003: America launches the War in Iraq with little or no support from the United Nations and other traditional allies like Germany and France, who both oppose the war.

- December 26, 2004: A tsunami follows a 9.3 Richter scale earthquake in the Indian Ocean and 290,000 people die in one of the greatest natural disasters in history. Ten months later, 75,000 people die in the Kashmir Earthquake.
- August 29, 2005: Hurricane Katrina inundates the iconic city of New Orleans. Between 1,300 and 1,800 people perish from Alabama to Louisiana in one of the worst natural disasters to strike the United States.
- January 21, 2008: Stock prices tumble internationally over fears about the United States' economy, set off by the collapse of the housing market and failures of banks in the United States and Europe. Consumer confidence in the banks and credit availability absolutely self-destruct. The United States and most of the world sink into a deep recession.
- June 1, 2009: The H1N1 virus (swine flu), the latest in a series of recent biological threats, is confirmed by the WHO (World Health Organization) as the first official pandemic since the Hong Kong flu of 1967–1968. Visions of the great flu pandemic of 1918 spark government and public anxiety.
- 2010: An earthquake in Haiti kills 100,000 people and completely decimates the country. North Korea threatens to start a nuclear war with everybody. WikiLeaks undermines the Western governments and their allies by posting confidential documents on the Internet for everybody to see.

For America, the decade 2000–2010 could easily be described as the "worst since" decade: the worst act of domestic terrorism ever and the first time a foreign power has successfully waged war on mainland United States territory since the War of 1812. We also dealt with the worst American wars since Vietnam, the worst pandemic since the '60s, the worst recession since the Great Depression, the worst national and international nonepidemic natural disasters since the San Francisco earthquake of 1906, and the worst financial scandals since the sleazy savings and loan dealings of the 1980s.

In addition to these "worst since" events, for the first time in history, the world watched through the eyes of modern technology (Internet, blogs, cable news TV) as events seemed to confirm our fears of what could happen when the shit does indeed hit the fan. During the Katrina disaster, for example, we watched 24-7 as a full week of chaos and mayhem went on right in front of our eyes. Perhaps a third of police and many firefighters and EMS personnel abandoned the city, many in their official response vehicles. The brave police and other responders that remained watched as residents formed gangs and roamed the streets, not only looting for food and essentials, but also feeding their greed with nonessential items. When lootable supplies were depleted in their own neighborhoods, they migrated to others. Those emergency workers who did respond found themselves under fire, and before long the military was called in by the tens of thousands to take control. Big, big lessons were learned here by the average person watching on TV, and a grim confirmation of some survivalist predictions unfolded right before our very eyes.

Even as I finished this book, the world was rocked by social-network-inspired rioters turned rebels bringing down long-term governments in the Middle East. Beyond the warm and fuzzy feeling we get when we think of democracy coming to these countries is the cold hard fact that the Internet in the form of social networking has now reached the capacity to topple stable governments, sending oil prices spiraling and prolonging the economic disaster we were just recently recovering from. And as I sit in my hotel room finishing the final draft of this very chapter, an 8.9 earthquake, the most powerful in Japan's recent history, kills thousands, sends a tsunami racing toward the West Coast, and creates potential nuclear catastrophes at five "earthquake-proof" nuclear power plants, an event covered from start to finish in fine detail by CNN and Fox.

No wonder Americans are nervous. The effect of this constant bombardment of bad news can't be overstated, and the public's trust in politicians, criminal justice, contract law, financial institutions, and Mother Nature herself is nonexistent. A ten-year war has dropped us to our economic knees, and a few hundred thousand disillusioned combat veterans are back, searching for jobs, health care, and homes. This is an enormous, righteously unhappy, well-trained army with the right to bear arms whose enemy seems to be the federal government. It doesn't take a genius to sense the potential threat. It would not be far-fetched to say that survivalism and the thought of having a safe haven from it all, a retreat, is now firmly established as a fundamental interest in the minds of most Americans.

During all of this, the inventory of survival, survivalism, and retreat-oriented books has spiraled. Add this one to the list. Hopefully you, the reader, will find this book to be a reasonable, rational, and simplified examination of what can be done by the average joe to prepare and manage a functional retreat.

Chapter 3

Retreat Strategy and Management

PLANNING

PLANNING IS THE KEY TO PREPAREDNESS, AND WITHOUT A PLAN, there will be no trip wire. Although this book contains information on retreat planning, readers are advised to purchase a book like *What to Do When the Shit Hits the Fan* and take note of the specific information on general disaster planning. If you have a retreat to incorporate into your planning, you'll need to factor in the following:

- When to retreat ("tripwire events" per Benson)
- How to get to the retreat—means, route, contingencies
- How long you may be at the retreat
- Who decides and what criteria are used to decide to leave the retreat

ORGANIZATION

Some retreats are organized with a single (usually patriarchal) leader, while others are more socialist in nature. Some are organized as democratic—sometimes dictatorial—group retreats. Group retreats often have a new age component and are sometimes referred to as intentional communities. They are usually founded

A polygamist colony built as a self-sustaining retreat in the remote American Southwest desert.

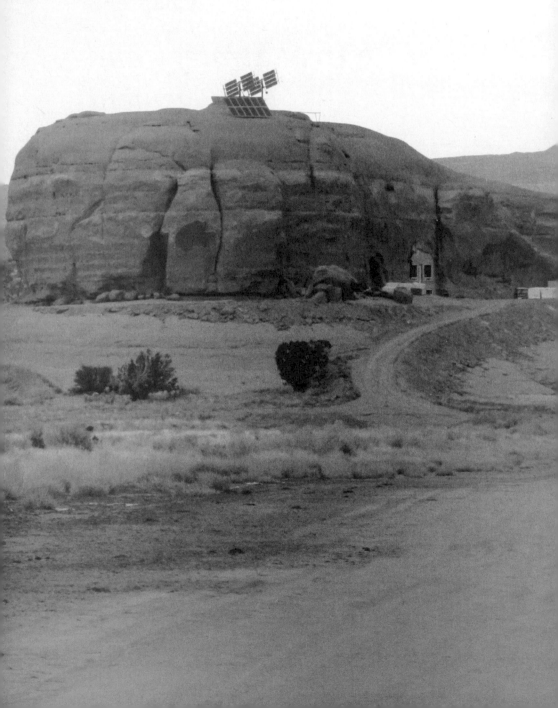

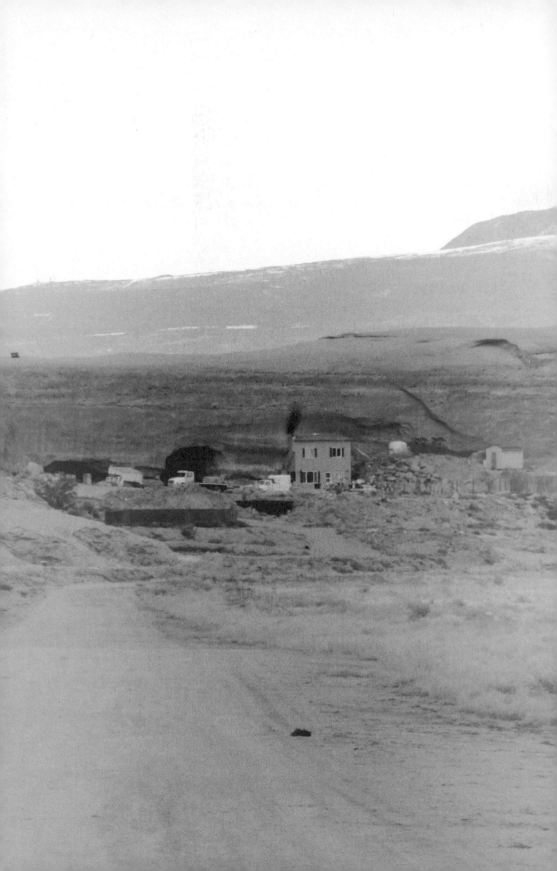

by individuals or families with similar interests—primarily family, welfare, politics, or religion.

Community retreats with a religious influence are sometimes called "covenant communities." Religious retreats are prone to failure for many reasons, including elitism, antisocial appearances, the tendency to set themselves apart while remaining highly visible, and the likelihood of blind compliance to radical leadership.

LOGISTICS

Logistics are a key component of preparation for long-term survival situations. Some of the key logistic elements (essential supplies stockpiled for survival and barter) are as follows:

1. **Long-term food storage**
    As C. W. Nelson of *Alpine Survival* says, "Food is king." The most common food supply goal seems to be a one-year supply, according to popular writers and primary proponents such as the LDS (Mormon) Church. It should be noted here that the LDS Church has been a longtime advocate of a one-year or multiyear emergency cache of food and essential supplies. This is the direct result of the Great Depression, but had its indirect roots in the long history of repeated interference and persecution by state and federal governments that eventually led to the Utah War, an event that bears some attention by survivalist groups. Individuals looking for some free practical advice on food storage can contact local church officials or the local congregation's Relief Society.

    How much you store is going to depend on several factors:

    -   Estimated duration of the crisis (a week? a year?).
    -   Storage space.

- Cost.
- Availability of supplemental food. As discussed later, even in dense urban situations, it's possible to grow something fresh and perhaps raise a few animals. See chapter 5 for farming ideas.

Most survival manuals have similar storage recommendations. Storage today is easy due to the proliferation of dried,

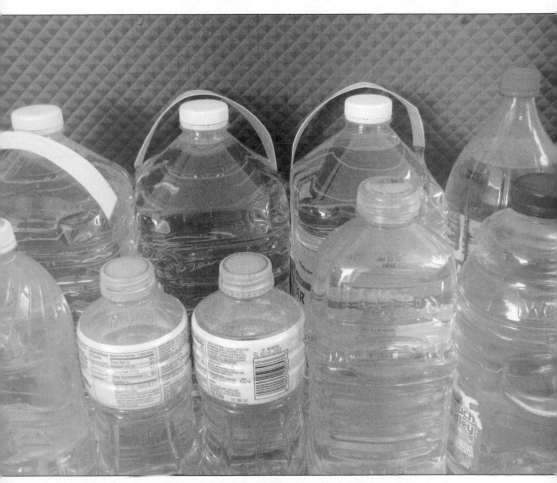

Building a stored water supply is easy. There's no need to stress about containers. Old water or juice containers can be carefully washed and refilled with water for storage.

freeze-dried, frozen, irradiated, and canned food products. Try to aim at providing about one and a half pounds of food per person, per day.

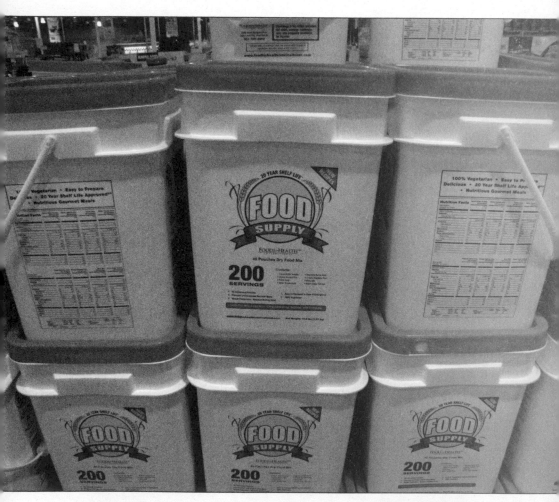

Among the maze of racks and aisles in a local Costco, I saw some amazing bargains for budding preppers and survivalists: vegetarian survival rations in a handy two-hundred-serving take-home bucket ($68), solar-powered ventilation fans, and Coleman 55-watt solar power kits that include a controller and 200-watt inverter ($217). Survival just keeps getting easier.

2. **Water**

   A gallon per day, per person for drinking, cooking, sanitation is the standard. Learn to harvest water, and make contingency plans for harvesting/filtering/purifying supplemental sources.

3. **Tools**

4. **Defensive weapons**

5. **Ammunition for hunting, self-defense, and barter**

   As will be noted later, common popular calibers of ammunition (.22 caliber, 9 mm, 7.62 × 39 mm, 12-gauge, etc.) are likely to become an excellent tool of barter if the time comes when currency loses its value.

6. **Gardening seed and fertilizer to supplement and extend food supplies**

7. **Medical supplies and the knowledge to use them**

8. **Fuel and/or sustainable forms of energy production to run vehicles and keep appliances and amenities functioning**

   If petroleum is your mainstay, plan on storing a gallon per day of compressed or liquid fuel. If you've got the ground space and the means, consider placing buried fuel tanks.

9. **Sanitation**

Obviously, these necessities are exactly what the marauding hordes are going to be looking for. They will want to feed their families too, and they'll do what they need to get them. Interestingly enough, alcohol (wine and spirits) are frequently listed as an essential logistical element. With the exception of the obvious uses as barter and tranquilizer, there actually seems to be little reason to include alcohol on that list, especially considering the historic tendency for alcohol consumption to make matters worse. Certainly, during social chaos and pandemonium, wine and cheese parties are not likely to be a priority. With that said,

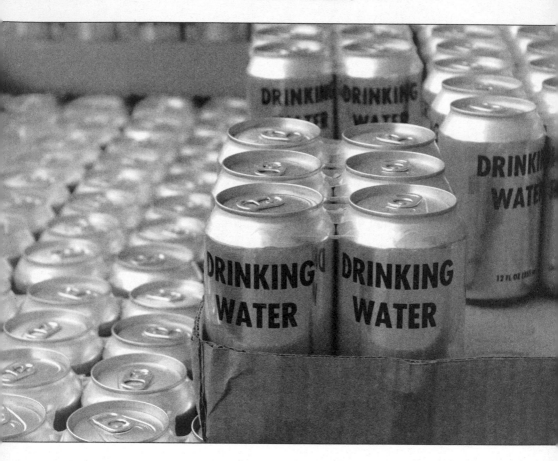

alcohol will certainly be on my personal list of consumable essentials.

Another consideration is caching. Many survivalist experts recommend caching additional supplies at separate locations that can be accessed if the group finds itself on the run or if they find that their main supplies have been pilfered. Captain Dave (www .captaindaves.com/guide/cache) has an excellent discussion on what/where to cache and how to locate and recover a cache.

The final word on supply and logistics: ALWAYS HAVE A CONTINGENCY PLAN AND ALTERNATIVE RESOURCES.

Networking

Many survivalists and preppers are staunchly against generating any kind of high-profile association that may draw attention to their retreats and preparations. This makes perfect sense to me. To modify a phrase from *Field of Dreams*, if you build it, and blab about it, they will come. Hungry, desperate people will target your supplies and all of the resources that you've worked hard on saving. If the zombies know you've got goodies, then they'll most certainly be there at dusk.

Other survivalists and preppers are convinced that the key to long-term survival is networking with other survivalists for support. An example of this is ANTS (Americans Networking to Survive). The website describes themselves as "a survival network comprised of individual preppers working together to provide other members basic supplies during disasters. This is done by forming supply chains between members locally and nationwide."

An important recent resource that is being used more often by survivalists and preppers is social networking sites (Facebook, Twitter, etc.). They can be used to network with persons with similar interests, but of course, care must be taken to limit the amount and type of information (intelligence) one makes available for the public to see.

Chapter 4

The Physical Aspects of a Survival Retreat

SELECTION CRITERIA

THE FIRST THINGS THAT NEED TO BE DETERMINED BY SOMEONE WANT-
ing to establish a survival retreat are

1. Purpose and
2. Location

PURPOSE
Will this be a short-term retreat, i.e., a prepper's haven, a long-term retreat for a last stand in an apocalyptic EOTW (end of the world) scenario, or something in-between? The main difference is the amount of logistical support that will be needed.

LOCATION
Let's start the discussion on location by defining three basic geographic locales.

Urban locations are in the city, within land densely occupied by buildings and other structures used for residences, institutions, and commercial/industrial sites. Urban implies buildings built high and more close together than in suburban areas and usually having more than one form of public transportation, i.e., bus, subway, rail.

Suburban locations are in areas on the outskirts of cities and contain structures that, on the average, are lower and farther apart than in urban areas. The population density is smaller, but the same services are available (school, health care, public works, fire/EMS/law enforcement). Some forms of public transportation are available, which are often in the form of commuter trains or buses.

Rural locations are usually remote from cities and characterized by large amounts of open space and contain a significantly less dense population. Structures are often farther apart, and services (schools, hospitals, etc.) are shared between communities. Public transportation may be absent altogether.

How does this make a difference? Many, if not most, survivalists are inclined to go for rural remote locations as a means of getting away from urban locations where their main fear is that they end up getting trapped with a million other people, searching for food, barter, and revenge. What many fail to see are the equal advantages of staying in urban or suburban areas for the purpose of blending in. As various survivalist writers point out, setting yourself out from the crowd may be a faulty strategy. In the animal kingdom, singling out a straggler from the pack is how predators identify their next meal. There's safety in numbers, especially if a shred of genuine law enforcement and public safety service remains intact. In analyzing retreats that ultimately failed to protect their occupants, one of the most common factors seemed to be that the group did not blend in to their surroundings. The second factor that they failed to take advantage of was the protection of the surrounding population, or more simply, the herd.

A second question to ponder when deciding whether to retreat in your urban or suburban home or to purchase land and develop a remote retreat is, if you're not living in your retreat

24-7, what makes you think somebody else won't find your retreat before you get there? In an EOTW situation, the roads, if not destroyed, will probably be blocked and patrolled by thugs. You won't be driving to your retreat, and it may take days, even weeks, to get there by foot. What if the zombies take over the retreat before you have a chance to flee there? Then the problem is compounded, and you have nowhere to go and only limited supplies on hand. Your new alternative, unfortunately, is to join those very hordes you've been so worried about. Now *you* are the living dead, and the retreaters and survivalists are hiding from you. In a practical and even a strategic sense, it's more logical to hunker down where you live, where you can blend in, and where there's still a smidgen of societal protection left available. If this isn't your plan, then consider keeping at least a seventy-two-hour kit on hand for each person in your party and a few nearby seventy-two-hour caches. Another decision you will need to make is whether to prepare a contingency retreat and contingency escape plan to get to your retreat if plan A fails. At the very least, some alternative survival locations should be designated in your plan.

So, let's say you've pinpointed which circumstance your retreat is destined to fit in. We'll examine the possibilities.

RURAL
Traditional survivalist wisdom dictates a retreat in a location with the following:

- Sparse population
- Plenty of water
- Arable soil
- Adequate solar or wind exposure for energy production.
- Good solar exposure for farming
- Defensible terrain

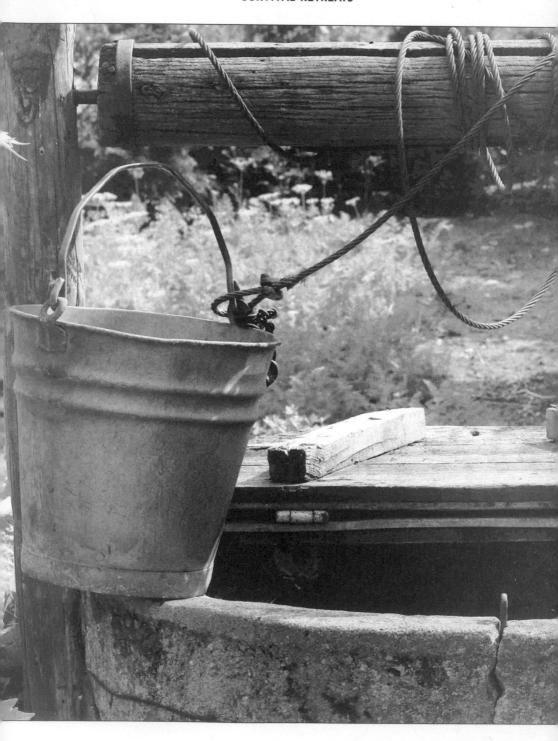

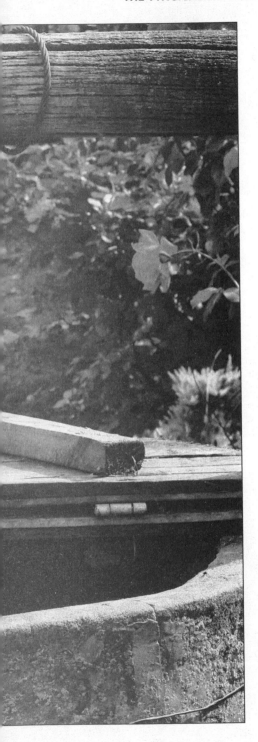

Additional preferences often mentioned in modern rural retreat criteria include the following:

- A distance of more than one tank of gasoline away from large urban centers.
- Locations not located along major lines of refugee traffic or major corridors of travel from urban areas. These would preferably be out of sight of major roads and highways.
- A location with definitive tactical advantages:
  o Remote, well off-road, and requiring lengthy hikes to approach.
  o High ground or terrain easily modified for tactical defense or escape and evasion.
  o And the ability to dig back into a hillside or into the ground forest canopy cover, as well as many others.

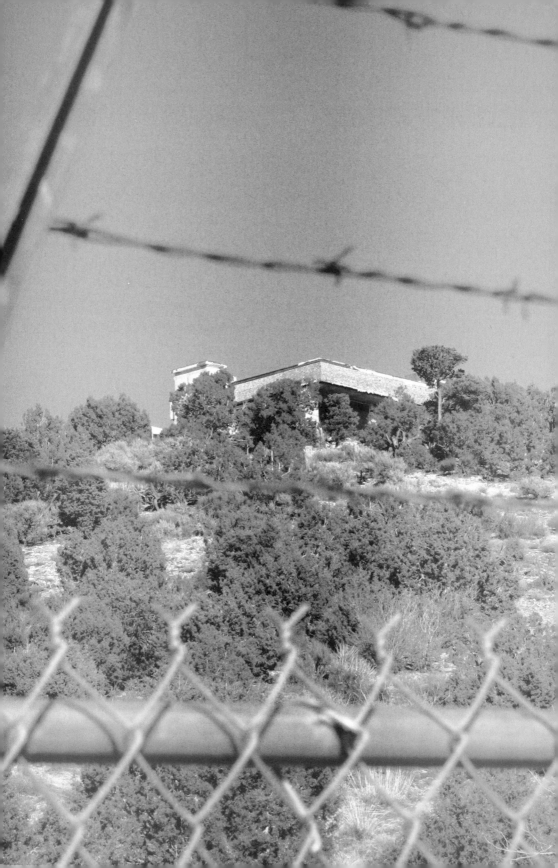

This is an off-road retreat home in a small Arizona town, ninety miles from the nearest urban center. It's located adjacent to several reservoirs, on easily defendable high ground with farmable soil, and has prime solar and wind exposure for energy production.

If this is an eleventh-hour retreat—a place to escape to when all hell breaks loose—planning consideration must be given to interim protection and transportation to the retreat or the whole concept becomes a moot point. An urban or suburban escape vehicle (a BOV or "bug-out vehicle") should be available, stocked with its own bug-out bag, the mechanical configuration and fuel capacity to get you where you need to go (4WD, motor home, etc.), and with enough supplies to maintain you and your group for at least as long as it takes you to get established in the retreat or find the next cache.

SUBURBAN AND URBAN

Retreating where you live or work is referred to as "bugging in." This may involve as much as turning the entire house, yard, or even an apartment into a self-sustainable fortress or as little as preparing to "shelter in place" in a single room. Shelter in place involves taking immediate shelter wherever you are, perhaps for just a few hours or days, and usually in a central interior room that is then sealed off from contaminants as needed. It normally has no additional defensive upgrades in terms of construction. However, a preselected shelter should have walls well secured to the foundation, wall studs strongly secured to the roof rafters, and large appliances secured with cable or metal stripping. An emergency stash (the seventy-two-hour kit) should be stored there, and well-planned shelters will include a means of communicating with the outside world (cell phone and two-way radio).

When you add the self-defense piece of survivalism, that simple single-room shelter becomes a variation of the "safe room" or "panic room." Safe rooms come in two flavors. The safe room FEMA recommends for protection against natural disasters, and the panic-room-style safe room designed to serve as a secure sanctuary modified to withstand an all-out assault. Safe rooms are new or preexisting, may be built above or below ground, and specifically are built or modified to withstand the devastating forces of nature or a deadly mob assault, depending on which flavor you choose. In simpler times, these were called "storm shelters," or were simple hidden rooms under the baseboards. In modern times, hidden basement rooms are still a viable option.

Safe rooms that meet FEMA standards for wind disasters are costly whether you buy the prebuilt versions or do it yourself. A well-made safe room is constructed by using wood and steel or reinforced concrete, welded steel, or other superstrong materials. It is usually built in a basement, on a slab-grade foundation, on a garage floor, or in an interior room on the lowest level. The room is anchored securely to resist overturning, and the walls, ceilings, doors, and all connections are built to withstand extremely high winds and prevent penetration by wind-borne debris. If built belowground, your safe room will also need to be flood-proof.

Panic rooms are also available prebuilt or can be do-it-yourself and are essentially a defense system rather than a reinforced waiting room. The most common choices for panic room locations in existing structures are large closets or master bedrooms with a bathroom. A large home with several floors might have a panic room on each floor. If you decide to use a room within an existing structure:

- Choose a windowless interior room.
- Make certain that the door system is solid. Reinforce existing doors or replace them with solid hardwood-core doors, and reinforce the wooden doorjamb or replace it with a steel one. Whether the room is DIY, prefab, or built with the house,

panic rooms usually have hidden entryways. Entryway doors are often made of steel and have mortise locks (built into rather than attached to the door) and steel doorjambs. If the door doesn't open inward, install security hinges or pin the hinges.

- Install a keyless dead bolt and consider multiple locks. High-end rooms might have a keypad-controlled electromagnetic lock. Complex lock systems might include a combination of keyed locks, keypads, and scan devices (fingerprint or retina).
- Stock it with at least a seventy-two-hour supply of essentials.
- Fortify or reinforce on all sides, walls, ceilings, and floors. Thick plywood reinforcement adds a small degree of ballistic protection, a significant degree of storm protection, and cannot be kicked through like sheetrock can. Additional measures might include wire or steel mesh and blast-proof Kevlar panels. Lightweight Kevlar and plastics can be used on wimpy upper floors.
- Consider including alarm systems and cameras.
- Windows, if there are any, should be reinforced and lockable, covered with a grill or bars, and adorned with heavy curtains and other view blockers.
- Include a communication system (cell, Internet, and radio) and an armory (weapons, a safe, and ammunition storage).

The panic room is a family protection system that is most likely to be used as a temporary retreat from home invaders where the family can wait, call for help, and stay in communication with the authorities. In a worst-case scenario, this is also a place to hunker down and make your last stand against the marauding zombie hordes that have surrounded you, penetrated your perimeter defenses, and entered your home.

Building a foolproof perimeter defense and an assault-proof panic room is no easy task and is certainly going to be easier in the suburbs than in urban areas, where the population is dense and residential properties are small and tightly packed. Even under those circumstances, though, some simple modifications can be made to the apartment or home that provide an early warning system and can turn a bedroom into a functional panic room. If modifying a small room within an existing structure, a reasonably secure room can be had for a couple of thousand dollars. A professionally designed, high-end room can cost half a million.

One last point on logistics: Having a retreat in an urban or dense suburban area doesn't necessarily exclude you from water sources or from agriculture to augment food supplies. Crops and herbs can be grown in plant boxes, parks, median strips, or even inside at the windowsill or under grow lights. Meat, i.e., rodents, small animals, and chickens can be raised in cages. Water is every-where in the city. It may be ugly filth, but unless it contains toxic chemicals, it can be filtered and purified.

Retreat Construction

A residence or dedicated retreat can only be entirely invulnerable and self-sustainable if defense and sustainability are designed and integrated into the structure as it is being built. Even so, it is very possible to defensively harden and to reach an acceptable degree of sustainability by making some modifications to your existing structure.

Making your home into a retreat does not mean destroying the comfort or the beauty of the structure. Also, it does not mean disrupting the primary use of the structure or the rooms within it. For instance, your bedroom will still be a bedroom, even if you've turned it into a safe room, and it won't have to resemble a '60s fallout shelter.

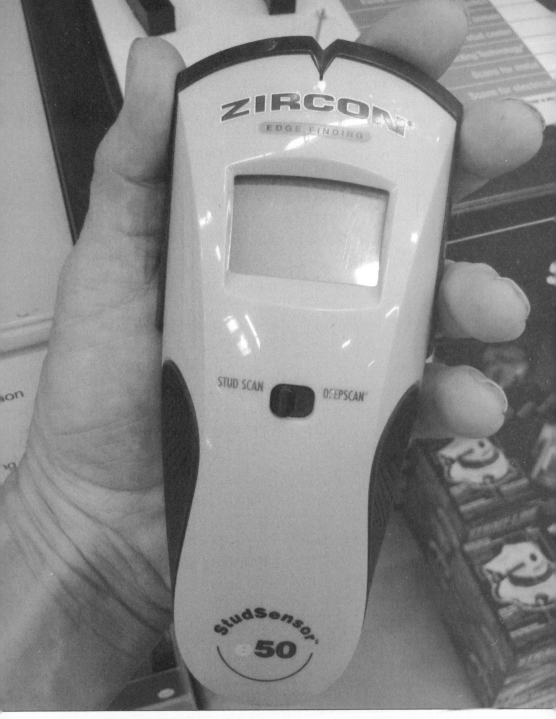

A stud finder is handy for impromptu window and door sealing to keep the zombies out. Nailing a plywood sheet to your drywall doesn't work. They'll just push it in. The plywood must be deeply nailed, preferably screwed, into the studs within the wall.

Commercially Designed, Prefab, Constructed, or Contractor Installed

First and foremost, let's remember who this book is written for: the 85 percent of the population that controls only 15 percent of the wealth. Commercial shelters and panic rooms are expensive. We're talking over six digits in most cases to add something on or to incorporate a retreat into a new structure. This is insanely more than the average American family can afford, and once again, protection becomes the exclusive right of the wealthy unless we can offer some reasonable and inexpensive alternatives such as those discussed later in this book.

Buyer should also beware of any purchases and go about buying your retreat as you would when you bought your own home. Building permits will be required in many, if not all, cases. This not only makes you highly visible to authorities, but also places you at their mercy for permission. You must also be aware that from order to installation can take months until it is completed. Nothing happens overnight, especially when building permits are required.

Where to Get More Information

Here is a list of good websites than can be used to educate interested readers regarding the ups and downs, ins and outs of commercial retreats and shelters:

americansaferoom.com

beehive.erikrowland.com (prefabs based on hexagonal modules)

delagostti-industries.com

earthshelter.com

f-5stormshelters.com
flash.org
formworksbuilding.com
fortifiedretreat.com
hardenedstructures.com
northwestsheltersystems.com
oism.org (see the egg-energy shelter system)
shelters-of-texas.com
survivalcenter.com
undergroundhomes.com
usbunkers.com
utahsheltersystems.com
variosafe.com

Typically, commercial shelters and retreats are made of rebar and concrete or welded and insulated steel, making an air- and watertight structure. Panic and safe rooms are available in steel and fiberglass.

Underground shelters can serve as retreats, disaster shelters, safe rooms, and even data storage areas. Undergrounds are often built from prefabricated steel or fiberglass structures incorporating an arched roof (tanks and cylinders) for increased ceiling strength. Both quality steel and fiberglass provide good corrosion protection. Undergrounds are usually incorporated within the construction of a new home. They're all buried, except at ventilation and access points, which are often hidden by landscaping or due simply to the fact that they lie beneath the ground and are interconnected to another structure (the home). Ventilation is

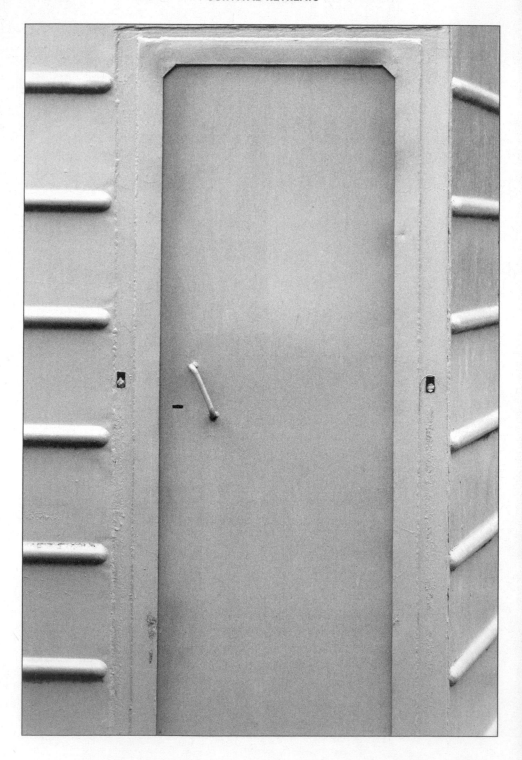

designed to provide a positive-pressure atmosphere which keeps out airborne pathogens and chemical gases. The air supply is typically cleaned through an NBC (nuclear, biological, chemical) filter, and the intake pipes are usually protected by a blast valve that prevents the overpressure wave from an explosion from entering the structure. The ventilation system should move air throughout the shelter in order to exchange carbon dioxide and oxygen. The air then exits the shelter via an outflow pipe that is protected by another blast valve.

A stand-alone shelter should have at least two ways in and out. There should be a main entrance and an emergency door or escape hatch, and should probably have primary and backup water and power supplies. More expensive underground shelter complexes are clusterable, may interconnect multiple modules,

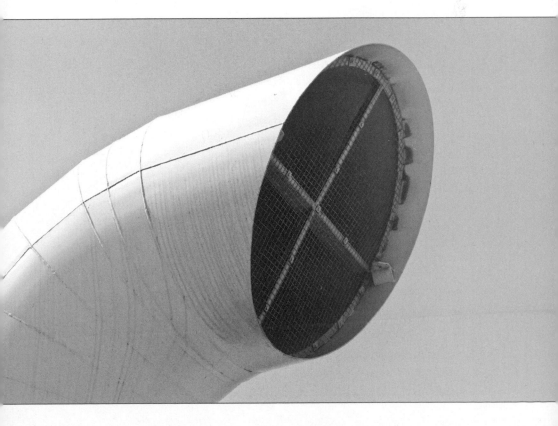

and may include a main shelter module, food module, water module, medical module, and utility (and armory) module. Each module can stand alone if other modules need to be cut off and interconnections can be made between neighbors for an underground community. Such shelter systems run somewhere around $300,000 or more per planned inhabitant, or about a million and a half for five people.

Basement shelters commonly have the same components but less blast protection unless structural changes are made. The advantage of doing a basement shelter is that power, water, and sewage utilities are already there, making it far easier to add onto an existing structure. Basement shelters also conveniently allow entry and exit without leaving the home.

Of course, there are DIY plans for a few hundred dollars, but even a shelter built from DIY plans is going to be expensive. A couple of interesting, less expensive concepts are the Hoag shelter system that uses a used fuel tank and the Sea Egg system, which can be seen on some of the websites at the end of the book.

Here's a list of things that are often included in a commercial shelter or retreat structure:
- Storage area for a large food cache (typically a month or year of food)
- NBC-filtered positive pressure ventilation system
- Emergency escape hatches or doors, lockable, with emergency manual opening mechanisms
- Lockable ladder entrance from overhead structures.
- Lockable air valves, water- and air-tight
- Specially formulated paint
- Wooden and/or carpeted floors
- Faraday cage protection against EMP (electromagnetic pulse)

Modifying Existing Structures

It's important at this point to remember that one of the key concepts in my series of survival books is that they are all written for the average person. Sure, it would be great to have a few hundred thousand dollars to drop on building a dream retreat or modifying the summer home to turn it into a retreat, but that's a pipe dream that belongs to the rich. One of the primary purposes of this book is to show what an average person can do to modify their existing residence to make it a safe and functional retreat.

It's my opinion that the key is passive home security, not booby traps and sophisticated arms caches. This slaps traditional survivalism in the face, but can be borne out by some precedence. The zombie hordes that attack your retreat are probably going to be just like any other criminals. A number of studies have indicated that violent criminals may average eight to ten points lower on IQ tests than noncriminals. Violent criminals may be more likely to be thwarted by complications blocking the approach. They tend to take the easiest path, and direct armed assault without obstacles is a lot easier than intruding into a retreat that's protected by a maze of security applications. In other words, spend more time and money on security and monitoring than on arms. Now that's not to say that you shouldn't arm yourself, actually on the contrary. After a zombie has wearily worked through the security obstacles, the idea of an armed conflict with an obviously intelligent and well-prepared opponent may be the final straw in his decision to call it off and find some other victim.

With that in mind, let's examine some possibilities. Even though this is DIY, to make a serious difference, you're going to have to spend hundreds, if not a few thousand dollars. Do it a little at a time. There's no hurry . . . for now the scavenging zombie hordes exist only in the minds of Hollywood types and science fiction writers.

Retreat Security

There are several external early warning systems that you should keep in mind.

1. Alarms

Most alarm systems are composed of multiple electromagnetic contacts placed on doors and windows that sense when they are opened and motion sensors (usually wall-mounted) that detect movement. Most sensors are PIRs, or passive infrared detectors, that respond to movement. Some systems include glass break sensors that sense the shock wave or sound of shattering glass. Systems can be wired, partially wired, or wireless, the latter being more expensive but easier for DIY.

   a. Alarm Services and Professionally Installed Alarm Systems

A basic professionally installed alarm system consists of a CPU (central processing unit, or computer), keypads—usually near the main entrance and in the master bedroom, where the entire system or just-selected zones are armed or disarmed by punching in codes—interior and exterior sirens and strobe lights, and door and window contacts. They will also include motion detectors, such as passive infrared detectors that sense human temperatures but not the lower temperatures of pets. Add-ons can include smoke and heat detectors, glass break detectors, panic buttons, remote operation devices ("remotes"), flood sensors, temperature sensors, carbon monoxide detectors, driveway alarms, and pressure mat alarms. Systems can either be wired or use wireless technology.

Another component of subscription alarm services is the service's own central monitoring station. Like the dish and cable networks, alarm companies make their money from selling you

services. That's how they can offer you the gear at such cheap prices, because they'll make it up with your subscription. The advantage of using an alarm service is that you can leave the area and
the company essentially house-sits for you. The central monitoring station will notify 911 if anything suspicious occurs, and some
of the more expensive services will even respond with their own
security team. What, though, can we expect from these subscription service providers during a widespread pandemonium situation when the grid has crashed? The monitoring station is likely
to be nonfunctional, and worse, there will be a group of gun-
packing, angry, unemployed security guards who know about
your alarm system and know precisely where you are.

Technology has progressed to the point that it is now possible
to have complete access to your professionally installed alarm
system from almost any location via the Internet. This allows fully
remote control and real-time monitoring. Don't count on this to
work when the shit hits the fan and the grid goes down.

A note of caution: unless your alternative power source is
wired into the electrical panel, any security device that runs on
house current should have a battery backup and must be capable
of being unplugged from the wall and plugged into the power line
coming in from the generator or inverter of the backup system.

b. Inexpensive Alarm Alternatives

Simple unmonitored systems can include any of the components
that a subscription-monitored service does with the exception of
the central monitoring station. These basic systems exist to warn
the residents and intimidate intruders.

Installation is simple:

- Window squealers
These are inexpensive electromagnetic contacts. A two-pack
at Wal-Mart was $6 at the time that this was written. The

detector is mounted on the door or window fixed frame, and the magnet on the door or window itself. Be sure to install the batteries before installation, and be careful with the alignment.

www.wikihow.com/Install-a-Door-or-Window-Magnetic-Detector

- Stand-alone motion-detector alarms and glass break detectors

Before installing these, be certain you know the detection range. Place them in a location were intruder movement is

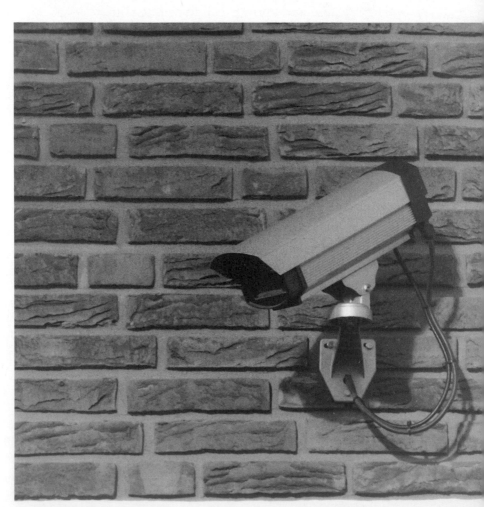

likely to be perpendicular to the direction the sensor is pointing rather than directly toward or away from it. Also, place them where they won't be adversely affected by heat, sunlight, or loose floor/wall vibrations. These are commonly placed at the front door, patio door, fire escape, and at other entry points or pathways around ground-floor dwellings.

2.   Cameras and Other Monitors

CCTV (closed-circuit TV) allows video images to be monitored or recorded from locations inside or outside the home. Some

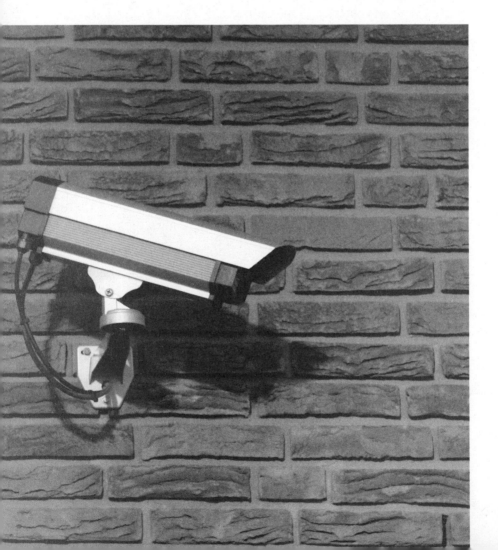

systems allow observation from remote locations via the web. CCTV systems can be wired or wireless. As with lighting and alarms, wireless systems are easier to install and don't require drilling holes in the walls. Like lights, solar-powered models are available.

A basic CCTV system consists of cameras, power supply, receiver, antenna (if wireless), monitor, and recording device. Many systems also include a remote control. Alternately, an inexpensive wired camera can be plugged directly into the AV input of the family TV, which then can serve as the receiver/ monitor. The salesmen are going to want to sell you a DVR to record the surveillance. This is nice, if you intend to use the device for everyday security. A video recording of burglars, intruders, or vandals is great to have when the cops show up. You can buy a separate DVR or you can purchase a DVR circuit board with cable ports to turn a computer into a surveillance center. When it comes to real bedlam and chaos, though, nobody's going to be interested in your videos, so for a retreat, a DVR is an unnecessary expense. Just patch the cameras directly into your TV or computer.

Cameras have become very inexpensive. A decent indoor/ outdoor color camera runs about $45, and includes a night vision mode which activates a bundle of infrared LED lights. More expensive versions might include motion-detecting IR which turns on the camera only when it detects movement.

Systems that hide the camera from view are called "covert systems." "Overt systems" are openly visible. Overt systems might scare a burglar away, but for a retreat, covert cameras seem like a better idea since marauders are likely to try to destroy any visible cameras.

With a few tools and the ability to focus on the instruction manual, almost anyone can set up a video monitoring system. The camera units are patched in to the safe room, the ops center, or other designated location where the resident(s) can observe intruders from a safe distance. This gives you time to get ready, gather some intelligence about your attackers, and call for rein-forcements.

3. Lighting

Obviously, intruders do not like being observed and often like to work under the cover of darkness. For this reason, it makes a lot of sense to install lights that illuminate all access doors, ground-level windows, the garage door, and any pathways that lead to or around the property. Light the front-entry doors and other important spots with two fixtures or a two-fixture lamp in case one fails. Overlap the lighted areas for complete coverage.

You must also consider energy consumption. Buy high-efficiency bulbs that get the brightest light (number of lumens) for the least power consumed (watts). These bulbs are not cheap, but they usually have an extended life. Also, what about your energy source? What sources will you have when the grid goes down? Batteries? Generator? Solar? Consider photocells for auto-matic on-off if you need all-night lighting. Motion-detector-acti-vated lights save energy and surprise intruders. Make sure that you mount them high enough above the ground that they can't be disabled.

Here are the steps for putting together an effective lighting system:

1. Sketch a simple floor and perimeter map (graph paper helps keep the scale accurate).
2. Identify areas around the structures and perimeter where light is needed.
3. For each area identified, determine the necessary lighting/detection zone.

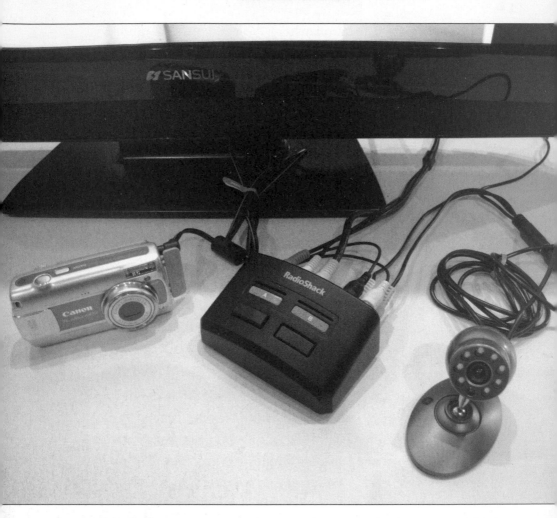

A simple flat-screen TV can be turned into a multiple-camera video monitor for under $100. Almost any low-voltage video source (a video security camera or even a simple point-and-shoot camera) can be used. This TV has two AV input ports. One port is plugged into a RadioShack AV selector switch that is plugged into two cameras. The TV's second AV input port is attached to the family's DVR or satellite receiver. With this setup, the family can casually toggle between a movie and two views of the intruding zombie hordes. The photo shows two very different cameras. On the right is a GE security camera with IR LEDs for night vision. Left is the family's old point-and-shoot digital camera with the auto shutoff function disabled.

- Doorways and small areas – 110 degrees
- Walkways and driveways – 150 degrees
- Side of house or garage – 180 degrees
- Corners, decks, patios – 240 degrees
- Sharp corners or large backyards – 270 degrees

4. Determine the type of fixture and the mounting height:
   - Ground-mounted floods – Avoid them. They're easy to destroy or dismantle.
   - High-output floods – These are mounted high for maximum coverage. They use mercury vapor or high-power sodium bulbs with extended life expectancy.
   - Adjustable twin-head floods – Double-fixture lights that can be aimed in different directions for maximum coverage and backup.
   - Residential lights – These will direct light downward, have shields, or have visors that can help prevent distant detection.
   - Area lights – Used to light large open areas.

A final note on lighting: don't aim your lights directly at your own ports of vision (the doorway, windows, etc.). The purpose of the lighting is to expose the intruder, not to blind the residents.

4. Dogs and other "alarm animals."

Dogs can function as an early alarm system and are, by nature, territorial. A deep, fierce growl or bark is intimidating, and every intruder knows dogs can be aggressively defensive. Large breeds associated with territorialism and aggressive defense include German shepherds, Dobermans, Rottweilers, bullmastiffs, pit bulls, and black Labs. Dark colors are more intimidating than light, although even light-colored or gentler dogs like golden retrievers make excellent alarm animals. Size matters in the case

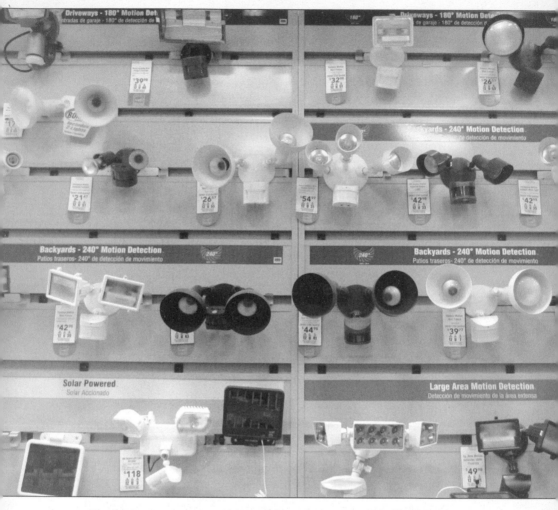

Check the light display at your local Home Depot, Lowes, or Wal-Mart.

of watchdogs; Chihuahuas and Shih Tzus don't inspire fear no matter how fiercely they bark.

Dogs need basic training skills and need to learn simple commands that will keep them safe and keep them from attacking innocent people. Teaching a dog to be aggressive is dangerous business that will get somebody hurt and could even get the dog euthanized. Most dogs bark naturally at intruders and need no training to function as an alarm, but they do need training to be able to recognize a threat rather than barking at anything and everything, which makes the dog useless as an alarm and annoying as a companion.

The program of training should include socialization to learn what's normal and what's a threat, basic command training, guard training using positive reinforcement (no hitting or chaining up for punishment), barking control (barks at visitors but stops on command), and property boundary recognition. It's also a good idea to give the dog access to the house and yard by installing a dog door that's low (too low for a reach-through) and just large enough for the dog but too small for a human.

Don't have a dog? Put up signs that will make intruders believe there's a dog, or, if you're rural or remote, consider alternative animals. The nice thing about alternative alarm animals is some of them can also help you with your sustainability plans by providing meat and eggs.

As kids who grow up on farms will tell you, geese are notoriously territorial and aggressive defenders of turf. They also have a loud and recognizable squawk. Geese are most effective in flocks with a single male. This eliminates fights between male geese. Geese will attack other animals, so pets and other animals must be segregated or trained to keep their distance.

Geese are less effective than dogs at patrolling boundaries. Some scratch feed thrown into the same location every day will keep them where they will do the most good. Other animals sometimes recommended for guard duty include donkeys and llamas. Visit this website for additional information:

https://web.archive.org/web/20140209060850/www.familyhomesecurity.com/alternative-guard-animals

Door Modifications

In urban and suburban settings, a formidable, threatening set of doors and windows is a real psychological deterrent. Intruders are likely to head down the block looking for easier pickings.

Here's some interesting reading: www.statefarm.com/simple-insights/safety/how-to-pick-a-door-lock-and-be-sure-its-secure

There are three primary ways intruders will get into your home (or retreat):

- Through an unlocked door or window
- Impact force (breaking the door or window)
- And prying (spreading the frame so the bolts don't extend into the strike pad) or jimmying

A full 83 percent of break-ins are successful by using one of these three methods, and there are even more ways to get through a locked door. The goal when modifying your door and window systems is to make it as difficult as possible, if not impossible, for an intruder to use door or window access. Perimeter doors, including yard doors and doors into garages or between adjoining living structures (apartments), should be equally protected. Also, remember that an unlocked garage or shed door gives your intruders cover.

Here are some key points:

1. Replace exterior hollow-core doors and the hollow-core door to your safe room (usually a master bedroom or large closet) with windowless metal doors or solid-core wood doors. By their very nature, hollow-core doors are lightweight, very wimpy, and easily destroyed with a shoulder, kick, hammer, or a shotgun. A hardwood core door puts 1.75 to 3 inches of solid

wood between you and the invader. Plywood, USB, or MDF wood composites are generally weaker and less plastic than hardwood. Avoid molded or decorative doors that have windows, mail slots, or thin-walled recesses that can be easily breached. Mail slots should be protected with a letter box cage.

Typical simple solid-core doors are 1.75 inches thick and inexpensive (and go for well under $100). Thicker doors may require modification or replacement of the frame and jambs, and are much more expensive. If you're seriously worried about the zombies blasting through your door with a 12-gauge, keep some liquid nails and precut ½-inch plywood on hand to bolster your door.

2. Make certain the door hangs properly and fits the frame well. If not, it will be easier for an intruder to break through or jimmy the door.

3. Exterior doors should swing inward to prevent the intruder from dismantling the hinge pin. Install security-type pinned hinges or hinges with nonremovable pins on all exterior doors that open outward. The hinge can also be "pinned" by removing screws from opposing positions on both top and bottom hinges and driving a nail into the holes so that the head sticks out just enough to stay within the drilled-out hole of the opposite side. When the door is closed, the head of the nail engages the matching hole and holds the door in place even if the hinge pin is removed. See these websites for a closer look: www.hardwaresource.com/security-stud-for-door-hinges .html
www.natman.com/type/security-stud-hinges-door-hinges

4. Reinforce or replace the doorframe or doorjamb. The jamb is the vertical portion of the frame onto which a door is secured. Most types of door fasteners and deadbolts extend into a recess in the doorjamb when engaged, making the strength of

the doorjambs vitally important to the overall security of the door. If the jamb is wimpy, basic deadbolts and fasteners can simply be bypassed by kicking down or body-slamming the door. It is possible to buy used doors, but be sure to reinforce the jamb as well. New exterior doors are commonly sold along with the doorframe. Usually the strength of the doorframe is proportional to the cost and strength or weight of the door. If you can afford them, metal security doors and steel jambs are a good option.

One way to reinforce an old doorjamb is to pull away the trim to expose the gap between the framing (usually 2 × 4s) and the doorjamb. Pack this gap with wood (scrap plank is fine) so that the strike plate screws go completely through the wood without a gap, then replace the trim.

Another easy way to reinforce a doorframe is to install a long metal strike plate with long screws that go deep into the surrounding wall studs. These plates are manufactured by several companies and most large hardware stores will stock them.

5. Speaking of the strike plate, it's usually the weakest point of the door system. Use security strike plates on all exterior entrances. The strike plate is mounted directly into or onto the doorframe.

The standard strike plate that comes with the door may only be cosmetic. Install a heavy metal strike plate or a strike box/faceplate combo with extra-long screws that go into the stud. Screws should be staggered so that they don't go into the same wood grain, causing the board to weaken or split.

The combination of warning systems and good doors will go a long way toward giving you the time you need to get inside, close the doors, lock the zombies out, and grab the armament. But what about those locks? And what about the windows?

Installing Multiple Locks

First, replace wimpy, nonlocking doorknobs with hefty outdoor locking knobs. This should be done on at least each of the exterior doors, including the garage and the door to your safe room. Knob locks are available with keys or as combination locks. Most locking knob sets incorporate a spring bolt lock, which uses a spring to hold the bolt in place and offers only minimal security if the door is on the outside of the jamb due to the ease of moving the bolt with a blade. Next, you should install an ANSI (or BHMA) grade 1 single-cylinder dead bolt that extends out of the door edge and into the frame at least one inch (that distance is called the "throw"). Longer throws severely limit the ability of an intruder to get inside by spreading the doorframe with a crowbar. A single cylinder has one keyhole on its exterior end. The other end is inside the structure and has a simple rotating handle or thumb-turn to lock and unlock the door.

Installation of a dead bolt sounds complicated to most of us, but it's actually a simple process of removing the old lock, reboring the hole, and installing the deadbolt. Reinforcing the strike is only slightly more complicated. The following website is a superbly illustrated, simple-but-detailed step-by-step description of how to reinforce a doorjamb and frame and install a new dead bolt lock:

www.familyhandyman.com/home-security/how-to-reinforce-doors-entry-door-and-lock-reinforcements/view-all

If your door has a window component, it can be shattered and the intruder can reach through and unlock the door. There are several possible solutions. The first is that the glass can be replaced with an unbreakable plexiglass or reinforced with a layer or sandwich of thick plastic laminate. Another option is to install a double-cylinder deadbolt.

A basic double-cylinder dead bolt has keyholes on both sides of the door. This is actually a fire hazard, especially if there are children living in the structure. As a result, most building codes do not allow double-cylinder deadbolts that don't have a thumb-turn. If you install these, make sure you leave a key in a fixed, permanent location in or near the indoor cylinder.

A variation of the double-cylinder dead bolt is the captured-key lock, which has a thumb-turn that can be removed from the inside cylinder, leaving a keyhole. The thumb-turn is actually the key, and it must be left in the lock at all times when anyone is in the structure. The same result can be obtained with a double-sided dead bolt by just leaving the key in place. Either way, these are hazardous. Imagine being caught inside without a key during a fire.

A variation of the standard dead bolt is the vertical deadbolt, which generally rests on top of the door. This is very resistant to jimmying. Other variations include single cylinders with removable thumb-turns, an exit-only function which has no external cylinder, and the mechanical or electrical push-button deadbolt. A rim-latch dead bolt is an alternative setup that locks automatically when the door is shut. It's great for a fast lock when retreating from the zombies, but it can easily lock you out.

A number of features are available for deadbolts. Saw-resistant bolts have internal pins that spin inside the bolt if someone attempts to saw through. Hardened-steel casings (the lock housing) make hammering and sawing even less effective. Beveled casings have rounded edges that make using a pliers or a wrench quite difficult. Hardened-steel anti-drill chips inside the housing destroy intruding drill bits.

Everyone in the group should know where the keys and spares are placed, and should practice the one-two-three, close-springbolt-dead bolt sequence so they don't forget one of the locks when they're in a panic.

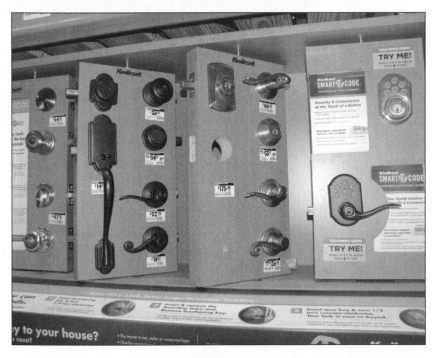

This image is of a lock display at the hardware store. Consider installing a lock pad (right side of photo). Most can be set to automatically lock when the door is closed, saving you precious seconds in a conflict situation. Opening the door takes a brief moment, and there's no key to lose or have fall into the wrong hands.

Keyless locks are also available. A simple changeable code opens the lock. They come with doorknob locks, deadbolts, and knob/dead bolt sets. Fingerprint locks are another, more expensive alternative.

Any additional locks that secure the door to the doorframe or floor (deadbolts, floor bars, foot locks) will add more strength to the door system. If a drop bolt or rim lock is used, it must be mounted on the door with through-bolts. Otherwise, a blow could cause it to separate from the door. A final option is to install a metal crossbar lock. They're ugly as sin, but can make a door nearly impossible to get through.

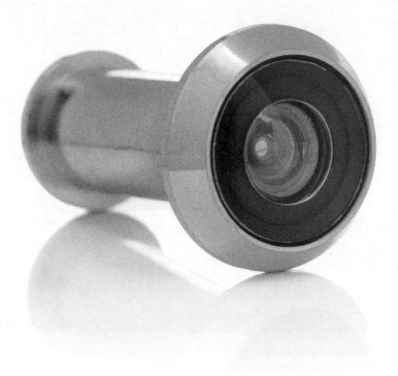

Wide-angle peepholes are a good way to be able to see the entryway without having to expose oneself. Most peephole viewers have a 180-degree horizontal field of view. They are usually made of metal and mounted at eye level. If there are short people or children in the structure, consider a second peephole at their level.

Some experts recommend installing a steel grid on the doorway because it can be both seen and shot through for defense. Grids or grills must be easy to open from the inside. Anchors that fasten the grill/grid to a doorway or window exte-

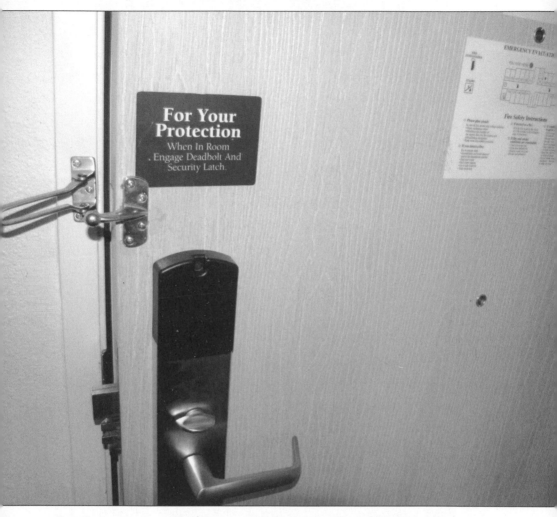

Good security in a budget motel: security deadbolt, flip lock, upper and lower peepholes, and a door wedge for good measure. Note that door limiters, flip locks, security chains, and surface-mounted door bolts are simple to install in the home but are generally weak and easily torn from the doorframe by a hard kick or body slam.

rior must not be easily unfastened from the outside (the zombies have screwdrivers and wrenches too). A storm door can be installed where an entry door is adequately recessed in the frame. A typical storm door has a half window and a lower panel

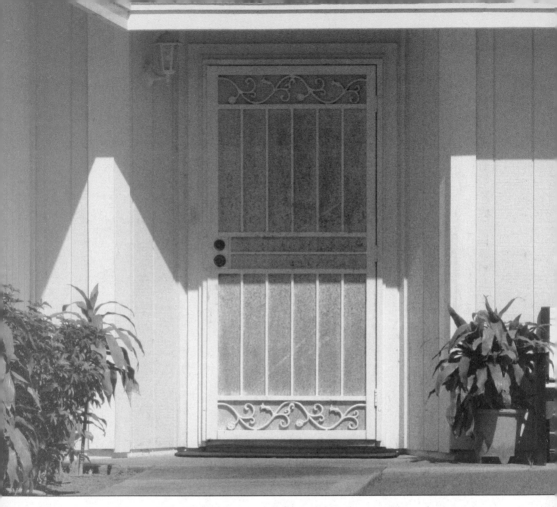

A steel security door over a solid hardwood core entry door is an adequate amount of door security for almost any neighborhood. Both doors must be properly hung to be completely effective, and must be installed with multiple locks and a reinforced jamb.

and may have a solid core. They are usually made to close automatically.

Other Types of Doors

Sliding Doors

Intruders love sliding doors, especially when they're in the back of the house and out of sight. They're often forgotten and left unlocked and are easily shattered with a rock, hammer, or bullet. The sliding panel should be mounted on the inside so that it can't be lifted off the track and removed from the outside. If it's not mounted on the inside, there is some security to be had by placing sheet metal screws through the upper track, just snug enough with the window that it can slide open but can't be lifted off the lower track. The door should most certainly have a strong key lock. You can also install a pin lock by drilling a hole completely through the sliding panel so a removable solid metal pin can be inserted to secure the sliding panel to the fixed panel. This type of pin lock can also be used to lock a double-hung sash window. A "Charley Bar" can be used to latch the sliding panel to the frame. Finally, the old dowel-in-the-track trick works nicely to keep the door closed or to allow it to open only as far as needed for ventilation.

French Doors

French doors, or any paired doors without a center post are not secure. Existing doors can be made more secure by installing heavy-duty vertical bolts and a quality dead bolt on the live door to secure it to the inactive door. Your other choice is to install ornate exterior security storm doors. These should have a heavy-duty two-inch steel frame, a quality deadbolt, and be prehung in a metal jamb.

Garage Doors

Install automatic openers or bolt-type locks on both sides (left and right) on the inside. Keep car doors locked, even in a locked garage. When going on vacation or when the marauding hordes attack, turn off the electronic opener system. As with other electronic security systems (lights, alarms, etc.), garage openers should have a backup battery and either a solar charger of its own or a way to plug into the backup power system.

Tilt-up garage doors are relatively solid and easy to secure with locks or pins. Automated retractable sectioned garage doors, on the other hand, may be made with panels held in place by flimsy molding and can easily be crushed or knocked in. Short of buying a stronger door (which is never cheap), there are only limited ways of reinforcing the sectional panels. Weighting the door with deadman anchors is one way to slow intruders down, but ultimately, the overhead door will be a very weak link in your security system. The door between the house and the garage is therefore critical.

Attic Doors and Hatches

Remove, seal, or lock exterior hatches or doors. Install a motion sensor in the attic and a screamer on the door if it can't be removed or sealed.

Key Management

Don't leave spare keys in the cliché spots, like under the doormat or in the flowerpot; everyone knows where to look. Use an external key lockbox with a combination code that is firmly mounted on a solid structure.

Reinforcing or Replacing Windows

Security windows come with shatterproof glass, are difficult to break through, and also extremely expensive. Full-on bulletproof glass is heavy and thick, requiring changes in the wall assemblies. Security or safety glass is made using one of two methods: tempering or laminating.

Tempered glass is made by treating the glass as it is heated and cooled to increase its tensile strength, making it hard to break.

When tempered glass does break, it snaps apart into rounded chunks. This is what the side windows of cars are made of. Laminated glass is made by putting a sheet of polyvinyl butyrol (PVB) in between two pieces of glass. When it does break, the vinyl layer acts like tape and holds the glass in place. Laminated glass is commonly used in car windshields and most security windows. Security windows are ideal, but for the "85 percent" group, a more reasonably priced and nearly as effective alternative is to cover your existing glass with a strong window laminate. If you have it installed, it will cost approximately $10–20 per square foot, which is almost as expensive as just going out and buying a new security window. But if you do the work yourself, it can be accomplished for as little as $2 per square foot; using glazing mastic to securely attach the glass to the frame will maximize the effect of the laminate. Storm windows (double pane) are more inconvenient to break through than single pane, and laminating both panes can make the window virtually bomb- and intruder-proof. Of course, die-hard security freaks are going to tell you it can't possibly be anywhere near as effective as real security glass. Skeptics should visit this YouTube site:

www.youtube.com/watch?v=j-i1MsVXFaA

Common window types include the following:

- Casement windows are made up of one or more sections or casements that open like a door. Hinges are located on one side ("side-hung") or along the top ("top-hung").
- Sash, double-hung windows have two vertically sliding "sashes."
- Awning windows have hinges along the top edge.
- Sliders are horizontal sliding windows with two casements or sashes.

Window opening mechanisms include hinges (usually butt hinges or friction hinges), tracks for sliding (double-hungs slide up or down, sliders slide horizontally), and tilts (casement windows that pivot). These are secured by various types of fasteners that hold or lock window sections together and stays that hold the window to the frame. Check them out, and if there's a weak point, replace them or supplement them with a backup of some kind.

Older windows need special scrutiny. Make sure the putty and glazing pins that actually keep the glass from falling out are intact; if not, simply redo them. Caulked and sealed wooden glazing beads are always a good idea.

Window security can range from locking fasteners and pins, to stay bolts and screw bolts, to multipoint mortise locks. Solid window locks that require a key and that secure component frames together are a good idea as well. The lock should be attached to the frame, not to the glass, and should be operated from the inside for safety precautions. In addition to being locked, windows should always be alarmed. Electromagnetic locks ("screamers") are inexpensive and effective. Install a rail clamp, dowel, or wood-block stop (screwed in if used in a vertical track) to allow the window to be opened a desired width for ventilation. Also, a motion-detector device could improve security if installed near each of the windows.

If you decide to go all out and "iron" your windows with grids, grills, or bars, remember that they must be fire escapable from the inside and not easily detached from their exterior side. With the exception of covering air conditioner holes, cages, grills, and bars are not generally recommended for residences. Motorized roll-down security shutters can be operated from the inside, but usually require professional customizing and installation, which can be very pricey.

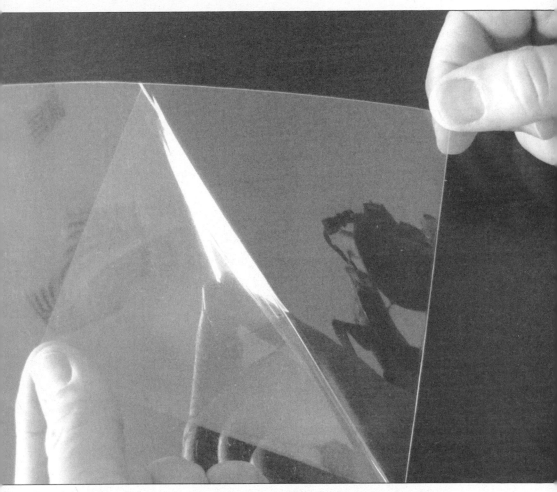

This photo is of laminate window reinforcement. Peel the backing off to expose the dry glue and apply to the window. Different thicknesses or multiple layers can be applied according to the threat (ballistic, explosive, high wind). The 0.009-inch and 0.011-inch thicknesses are the most commonly applied to residences and small businesses. The 0.003, 0.005, 0.006, 0.007, 0.014, and 0.020 are also available.

Skylights

Upper-floor windows and skylights should be equipped with locks, alarmed, and reinforced with safety laminate.

Curtains

Heavy curtains keep intruders from being able to see into the structure or room. They'll keep them from getting a clear shot of you with a weapon. You'll know where they are, but they won't be able to see you. Even if they do manage to get through the window, there's no telling what terrors you have waiting for them beyond those curtains.

Communications

In a simple seventy-two-hour-style disaster incident or a panic room scenario, a telephone is going to be the most important piece of communications equipment you will have. Telephone service will not be down for long, and the days where an intruder can cut your lines is behind us now that we're all using cell phones and as other alternatives are now available (like Internet telephone services such as Skype). If your retreat or room is too remote or armored for reliable cell service, get a buried phone (POTS) line, an intercom system, or an alarm button directly connected to 911 dispatchers or to a commercial security provider.

A bit of coaching is warranted here: In a typical home-invasion crime, traditional wisdom says that once you make contact with 911, you stay on the line as the event goes down. This allows you to be reassured by the dispatcher and to continuously relay updates to the responding authorities. Soundproofing the room or structure keeps intruders from hearing your conversations on the radio or phone, but it also limits your ability to hear early intruder warnings. However, if you're planning for a long-term, shit-hits-the-fan disaster situation resulting in widespread pandemonium, the cell and dish network towers are just as likely to be down as any other part of civilization's infrastructure; and don't forget, there is such a device as a cell phone jammer. In the end, a good old-fashioned radio may still be your best bet.

There's a lot to know about communications. The first book in this series, *What to Do When the Shit Hits the Fan*, covers this topic in greater detail.

What follows is a ten-point summary of the fundamentals.

1. Prior to and during a major disaster, most of the population will get their information and news from broadcast or cable TV, radio, or the Internet. These sources are easily corruptible and in a pandemonium-styled event could quickly become quite unreliable. The Emergency Alert System (EAS) broadcasts information and instructions via TV and radio stations. Also, the National Oceanic and Atmospheric Administration (NOAA) Weather Service Radio System will be a source of all-hazard information. Many FRS, GMRS, and ham radios come with preset NOAA frequencies and may also come with an encoder that automatically alerts the user when information is being broadcast.

2. Residents in remote or rural areas or who are located in other countries may have to rely on local resources for updated information. Look at the local (county or state) emergency plan and see how authorities plan to communicate emergency information to the public.

3. Keep a battery-, crank-, or solar-powered AM/FM/shortwave radio in your home and workplace emergency kits. Make sure you have extra sets of batteries as well.

4. Family and business associates might be dispersed. Make sure you have clear plans ahead of time for how you'll be able to contact each other during an emergency.

5. The traditional phone system, referred to as POTS (plain old telephone system), is powered through underground cables or the wires hanging from telephone poles. They will work during emergencies, as long as the lines aren't cut and stations are still functioning.

6. Cell phones rely on radio waves between the phone and the cellular tower. The radio channels can be oveloaded, and service can be affected by power outages at local servers or by destruction of relay and cell towers. Turn off your cell phone when it's not in use to conserve the battery.

7. Satellite phones transmit through low-orbiting satellites. They don't work well indoors without an external antenna dish. Also, they are heavy and expensive, and the system is not disaster-proof.

8. Wireless radio systems:

   a. Each country has its own electronic communications agency. In the United States, it's the Federal Communications Commission (FCC), and it assigns radio frequencies according to function.

   b. Radio signals, like all electromagnetic radiation, usually travel in a straight line. However, at low frequencies (LF, under three MHz), signals may partially follow the earth's curvature, thus allowing AM radio signals in low-noise environments to be heard well after the transmitting antenna has dropped below the horizon. Also, frequencies between 3 and 30 MHz (called high frequencies, or HF) can be reflected by the ionosphere, thus giving radio transmissions in this range a potentially global reach. But at higher frequencies (VHF and UHF), neither of these effects applies and any obstruction in between the transmitting and receiving antennas will block the signal. This applies to commercial FM broadcast radio, broadcast TV, cell phones, Wi-Fi, FMRS, GMRS, and MURS radio. The ability to visually sight a transmitting antenna roughly corresponds with your ability to receive a signal from it. This propagation characteristic is called "line of sight."

In practice, this varies, depending on the exact frequency and strength of the transmitted signal. Low-powered transmitters (FRS, GMRS, MURS, and local Wi-Fi) can be blocked by trees, buildings, hills, or even heavy rain and snow. Even the presence of objects not in the direct line of sight can also interfere with the signal. Reflected radiation from the ground can hurt the signal as well, though this effect can be reduced by raising the antenna farther above the ground. The resulting improvement in signal is referred to as *height gain*.

c. Getting licensed. FRS, MURS, and CB all run on low power and are extremely limited by line of sight. Their advantage is that they don't require a license and they are exceptionally inexpensive. FRS and GMRSs have the added advantage of multiple channels with multiple privacy codes. GMRS are slightly more powerful and do require a license, but don't require an examination. In all countries, amateur radio ("ham") licensing requires an examination to prove that the user has the knowledge of basic radio electronics and of the communication rules and regulations. In return, hams get more frequencies (larger "bands") and can use a much wider variety of communications technologies at substantially higher power—up to 1,500 watts (compared to half a watt for FRS).

What's the real advantage of basing your communications planning on radios? Well, when the shit hits the fan, radios will still function when nothing else will, and nobody can turn it off except the user who's listening.

d.   Setting up. Those CB, GMRS, and FRS walkie-talkies you see at the truck stop and hardware store don't require much of a setup. Take them out of the package, put in some batteries, and start communicating.

Mobile stations and base stations do take some preparation. Always have your mobile radio installed in your BOV by a professional. If you want to be able to use your mobile as a base station, get some detailed advice or have it done by a pro.

When installing a radio in your home or building, follow these steps for a comfortable and safe station:

1.   Dedicate a desk or specific area for the radio, hopefully at the command post.

2. You'll need access to the outside for the antenna and ground wires. Ground it as instructed in the installation manual.

3. Give the radio proper clearance from the walls for ventilation.

4. Use earphones to minimize noise and to keep intruders from hearing your conversations.

5. Cover the radio when not in use to protect it from dust.

e. Making contact. Here are standard guidelines for using two-way radios:

1. Monitor the frequency (a.k.a. channel) before transmitting.

2. Plan your message before transmitting.

3. Press the PTT (push-to-talk) button and briefly pause.

4. Hold the microphone two to three inches from your mouth.

5. Identify first the person being called.

6. Acknowledge transmissions directed to you.

7. Use plain English. Ten-codes and CB jargon confuse everyone.

8. Profanity is still illegal.

9. Reduce background noise as much as possible.

9. Data systems. Data is information, which includes text, numbers, and pictures. Devices used to transmit data include desktop and portable computers, fax machines, and "smartphones" (the combination of a PDA and a cell phone). Fax machines use phone, Internet, or radio services to send printed or illustrated

data. E-mail is message (text) data that's transmitted over wireless and landline systems.

Retreaters and preppers planning on using notebook computers and smartphones as their primary communication and navigation devices should remember that computer-accessed technology will not be available if power sources are knocked out or if the servers are damaged. E-mail, texting, and all those smartphone apps are lower-tier devices, subject to failure of other tiers: power supply, landline or wireless systems, servers, etc.

10. Primary and backup communication systems. Some thought should be given to continuity of communication. Right now, your primary means of communicating are your phones (POTS and cell) and your computer (Internet). These systems will very likely be overloaded, destroyed, or otherwise unavailable during a major disaster, leaving you with no way to communicate with the outside world. Therefore, radio is your answer.

Power and Other Considerations

The following considerations are mentioned here because they may or may not, depending on how complex your retreat is, lead to additions or modifications of existing structures, or may require some close attention when designing new structures. The two earlier books in the series, *What to Do When the Shit Hits the Fan* and *Living Off the Grid*, are recommended volumes of reference for a simplified look at alternatives for power and light, heating and cooling, and so on. *The Urban Homestead*, by Coyne and Knutzen, is also an excellent source of information and ideas.

Power basics

Most large or complex retreats will be powered by generators (which makes fuel an enormous bartering tool). The "gen" will probably be wired directly into the house or compound's current circuit board. It may be a backup for, or an integral part of, a multisource self-sufficient power system that could include solar and wind power generation and a huge battery bank. There are a lot of considerations to keep in mind. If you're planning on using a generator, pay close attention to the hazard of carbon monoxide poisoning. Generators will require self-containment or exterior placement. In the long term, wind and solar power may be the best solution; but if solar and wind are the major components of your system, be aware that a single bullet or a chunk of flying debris can pulverize your big panels or your wind turbine. You must always make sure that you take the proper precautions to protect them. For instance, amorphous and some other solar cells will still function with acceptable efficiency when overlaid by shatterproof plexiglass. Cables are better protected when they're buried. All in all, make sure you always protect the system.

Whatever technologies are chosen, they absolutely must be hardy and simple to maintain. Imagine a complex, commercially installed system breaking down after some widespread catastrophic event. Chances are there won't be any electricians available to fix it right away. Will you be able to do it yourself?

Also, you must maximize the efficiency of your system by learning to conserve energy and by using passive heating and cooling concepts that use the energy of the sun and wind to heat and cool without first changing it to electricity.

Solar power 101: The Fundamentals

- There are two types of solar energy systems. The first collects the heat produced by the sun's energy, warms air or water

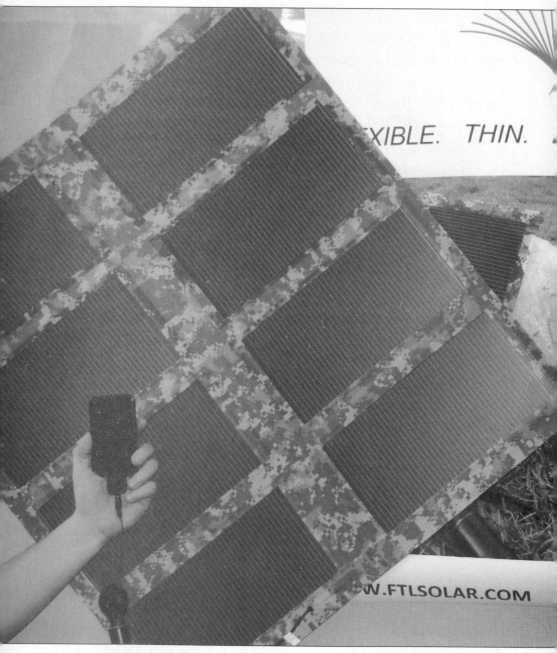

Fold-up, flexible solar cells that will not shatter and continue to work, even if pierced by a bullet.

within it, and then circulates it to heat a home or provide hot water. The second uses panels of solar cells to absorb the sun's rays and convert them to electricity, which is then used to run lights and appliances.

- Solar arrays are a cluster of panels, which are groups of photo-voltaic cells that convert sunlight to electricity. The bigger the array of panels, the more power (watts) it produces.
- Panels face the sun (southward in the Northern Hemisphere), unobstructed and tilted at the proper angle to get the most light energy.
- Some panels can be integrated into the structure as roofing or siding. Other recent technologies have produced soft folding panels that can be rolled up and carried wherever they are needed.
- Solar panels produce DC electricity (like the electricity in your car). Some tiny appliances can recharge or run directly off the panel, but most systems send the DC into a battery bank for storage. It's possible to run DC appliances directly off the batteries, but it's simpler and cheaper in the long run to plug an inverter into the battery bank. The inverter changes DC to AC (the type of current in your house), allowing the use of normal AC appliances.
- The question now is "what's involved in producing AC power?"
  - PV panels gather the sun's rays and convert them to electrical energy.
  - The electricity is sent to a battery bank via a charge controller (a device that prevents overcharging and voltage leaks in the batteries).
  - In the battery bank, the electricity is stored in "deep cycle" batteries, like marine batteries, as opposed to "shallow cycle" batteries, like those used in cars.

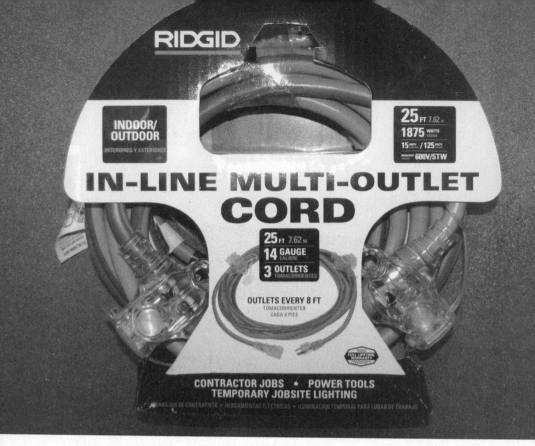

A properly rated multioutlet extension cord with outlets every 8 feet makes bringing the electricity indoors from your power system relatively easy.

- When it's time to use the stored electricity, an inverter changes the DC to AC. Power cords can be plugged directly into the inverter, or the inverter can feed a power panel that distributes the AC through the home.
- Other parts of the system will probably include the following:
  - Fuses and safety disconnects that prevent electrocution, short circuits, and fires. In very small systems, the safeties built into the inverter, appliances, and extension cords may be adequate. Larger systems will need more protection.

- Properly rated multiplug extension cords, preferably with circuit breaker mechanisms to protect from overloading and shorts.
- Any system, large or small, plugging directly into the existing house electrical panel should always be approved or contracted by a licensed electrician.

This is the Coleman 3-panel 55-watt solar power kit. Two kits will give the buyer 6 panels and enough spare parts (including controller, inverter, cables, and panels) to keep the system going for a couple of years. Four panels can easily be rigged to produce a portable 72-watt system. Four high-capacity deep-cycle marine batteries can be added to the system for about $300, and another $100 buys an inverter powerful enough to run a small refrigerator, air conditioner, or small heater. Bring the power into the home with a properly rated circuit breaker extension cord ($50).

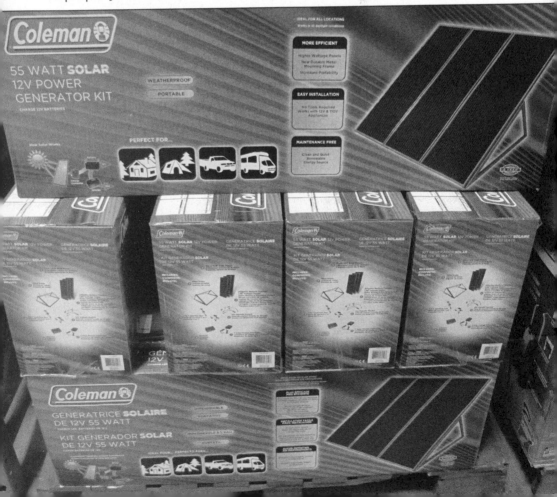

- A grid-tied system has enormous advantages but can be painfully expensive. For survivalists, the question remains, "why tie into the grid?" After all, if there is no infrastructure in the survivalist future, tying into the grid would be futile.

Wind Power 101: The Basics

- Harvesting power from the wind is very difficult unless you have the space and location to mount the turbine at least thirty-five feet above the nearest building. Wind power, therefore, is most pertinent to suburban and rural retreats.
- A microturbine can produce several hundred watts.
- The combination of a small turbine and a solar array ensures the continuity of production and storage of electricity without having to start the generator. On a good day, power is produced by the sun. On a bad day, it's produced by the wind.

On the other end of the scale are the simple power sources for short incidents. Battery operated LED lights or hand-cranked lights (some with mini solar cells, radios, and phone chargers) are now available in most hardware stores. There are even passive solar devices that can cook food, heat water for a shower, warm a room, and dry clothes.

Air Circulation

Air circulation will be a consideration in panic and safe rooms, many of which are made to be airtight and temperature-controlled. Passive ventilation measures might include static ventilation holes covered with a grill or active ventilation may be provided on a small scale using solar-powered fans (attic fans). Ventilation systems may include separate air filtration systems, which will protect against biohazard materials, dummy vents to throw off intruders, and individual PPE (personal protective

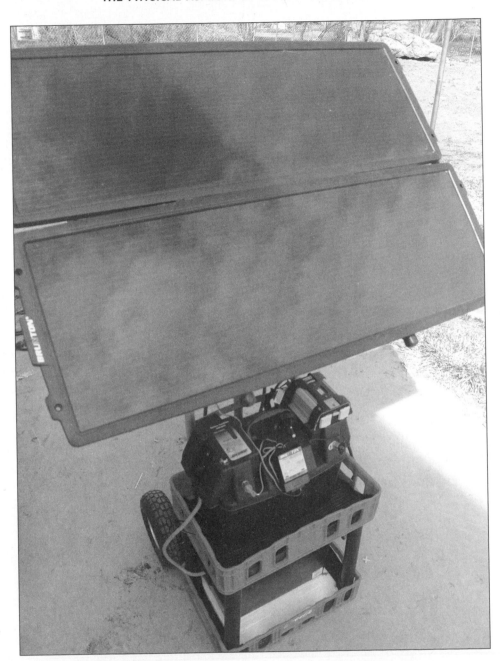

This image is of a 30-watt solar power system with a 400-watt inverter and 2-battery bank on wheels. It costs approximately $400, depending on where you purchase the components, and will run a computer and an electric blanket or low-watt fan for hours.

equipment) such as gas masks. Expensive retreats or panic rooms might have a filtered fresh-air system or even a sealed rebreather system with its own oxygen supply. Readers should note as they research air systems that "air" is not the same thing as "oxygen." Generally when we talk about an air system we're referring to a supply of "room air" which normally contains 21 percent oxygen. When we refer to an oxygen source, we're talking about oxygen tanks or an oxygen generator that supplies high-concentration oxygen for mixture with old room air.

Plumbing

Plumbing is the next consideration. Hopefully, the plumbing will continue to run during an emergency, but when the tap water becomes contaminated or ceases to flow, the prudent prepper or retreater will have a contingency supply of water stored on site, as well as some form of backup sanitation system (portable toilets, etc.). High-end retreats and most rural retreats will have their own independent plumbing and septic tank systems.

Chapter Summary – The Bare Essentials

In summary, here's the bare essential list of to-do's to prepare your grounds to function as a retreat:

1. Exterior Doors
    a. All exterior doors and the garage door are solid hardwood or metal clad.
    b. All entrance doors have both a keyed knob lock and a dead bolt.
    c. The doorjambs and frames are reinforced.
    d. The entrance door has a wide-angle peephole.
    e. Glass within thirty-six inches of the door is reinforced with security laminate or completely sealed.

    f. Security hinges or pinned hinges are used if the door opens out.

    g. Spare keys are not kept under a doormat or planter.

2. Windows and Glass Doors

    a. All are reinforced with security laminate.

    b. Safety locks are used that allow up to six inches of ventilation while still being locked.

    c. All are alarmed with electromagnetic contacts ("screamers").

    d. Sliding glass doors have a keyed lock.

    e. A pin or bar is used to prevent sliding doors from being forced open.

3. Outside

    a. Shrubs and bushes are trimmed so they cannot be used for cover or are removed completely to expand the visible perimeter.

    b. Each outside entrance is illuminated.

    c. Motion detection lighting is installed at all entrances and pathways.

    d. Gates, garage doors, and shed doors are always kept locked.

    e. A contingency power source is available to run security and other essential appliances.

4. A dog aids in intruder detection, and a weapon provides active defense when it's necessary.

5. Food and water for a predetermined length of sustainment is stored and/or cached, supplemented by farming that is already in progress and materials that are on hand for water harvesting.

Chapter 5

Food Sustainability and Supplementation

FARMING

By definition, retreats are supposed to be largely self-sufficient. So, like it or not, a real retreater is going to have to be a farmer as well. Unfortunately, farming is not something that can be learned on the spot. You can't have seeds hanging around in storage for years and then suddenly expect them to grow for you if you've never done any farming before. There are a lot of good websites with helpful suggestions. Start with this one and see what else you can find:

www.thespruce.com/container-gardening-4127755

There are many good books on the subject. One of the best is Coyne and Knutzen's *The Urban Homestead*. Much of what follows is influenced by that manual, and the author highly recommends it as part of the urban or suburban retreater's library. Most readers, after all, are urban and suburban dwellers with limited soil sources and very limited farming experience. Aside from teaching you how to grow your own food and raise your own animals for meat and dairy, Coyne and Knutzen's book contains information on urban foraging, and over seventy pages are dedicated to methods of preserving the harvest. Another thirty pages describe in-depth water harvesting techniques.

Below are some basic concepts of farming for foodsupplementation. Although these apply specifically to limited-soil scenarios, the same basics apply to farming on a larger scale.

1. Basic principles:
   a. Grow only what you can use. It will save you money and farming space.
   b. Develop a clean soil resource.
   c. Use more water, but do it less frequently.
   d. Do not expect any miracles. (Remember, Rome wasn't built in a day.)
   e. Keep constant notes as you never know when they'll come in handy.
2. If you have no access to ground soil, grow food in containers on patios, roofs, balconies, or indoors where they will get enough sunlight. You can also look into hydroponics and vertical farming. Maximize the growing space in all directions (string or wire trellises, etc.). Food crops need six hours of sun, direct or reflected, each day. If only inside space is available, place containers next to windows and supplement with artificial light.
3. Give priority to fruit-bearing plants (beans, peas, tomatoes, melons, cucumbers, squash, etc.).
4. Build soil in these ways:
   a. Compost all yard and kitchen waste and use as soil. Composting occurs when organic waste is broken down by microbial processes. When the process occurs on the forest floor, it's called mulching and the product is mulch. When the process is carried out by humans using pits or bins, it's called composting and the product is called compost. The resulting material can be used as fertilizer.

Efficient composting requires careful sorting and mixing of proper ingredients. Compost needs a good supply of nitrogen-rich vegetable waste (called greens), which includes scraps from the kitchen, grass and weed clippings, fresh leaves, and even coffee grounds. It needs a nearly equal supply of carbon-rich materials (called browns), which include straw, bark, wood chips, sawdust, dry leaves, and shredded newspaper. Don't add any bones, meat, fish, oils, dog waste, or dairy products.

Compost radiates heat if the nitrogen–carbon ratio is good. The warmth indicates that the aerobic bacteria, worms, and fungi are all doing their job. When the process is nearly complete and it's ready to be used as fertilizer, the compost will be cool.

Keep an eye on air and moisture levels. The microorganisms need air to work their magic, so be sure to mix it up and include some wood chips or straw to prevent vegetable products from clumping together and to keep the ventilation process going. The mixture should be damp but not wet enough to drip from the bottom.

The end result is a light, soil-like material called humus—a highly nutritious topsoil that can be spread over vegetable gardens, lawns, fields, and around trees.

b. Use mulch (leaves, etc.) to protect and build soil. Mulch holds in moisture, slows weeds down, and stabilizes soil temperature. Fall leaves, wood shavings or small chips, straw, pine needles, corn husks, and lawn clippings can all be used as mulch. Lay down a healthy cover around plants, about five inches deep. The mulch will break down and thin and can be replenished annually with fall leaves.

c. Be creative in finding or building places to grow your crops, preferably where they can get good sun exposure.

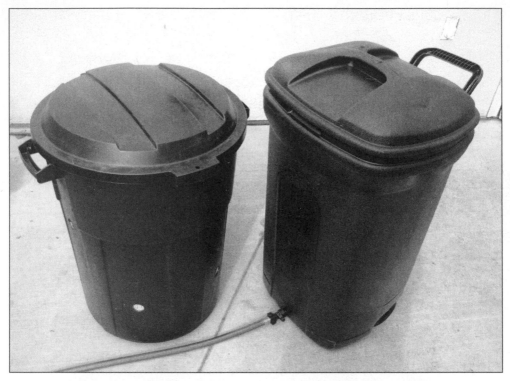

Tub Science at work. On the left is a composter made from a thirty-three-gallon garbage can. There are many quarter inch holes drilled into the can on the sides and on the bottom. The larger holes are screened and provide additional assurance that the mixture is getting enough air. To mix the contents, the container can be tipped and rolled every couple of days or weeks. Don't wait for the end of the world to start composting. These bins take three to four months for a family of two to fill and another six months or so to become humus, so a second or third bin will be needed. In urban areas "browns" may be scarce until the fall leaves are distributed by the wind. In your storage, you'll want to start keeping old newspapers and save your sawdust.

On the right is a thirty-four-gallon wheeled garbage can fitted with a cheap hose valve fixture to allow the hose to be turned on & off. When full, this contraption will run fifty feet of downslope soaker hose or a simple ring sprinkler at a drizzle for a couple of hours. Fill the can by using rain gutters or collector tubs. Otherwise, keep the lid on to prevent mosquito breeding. Filtered or treated gray water can also be used to help fill the can.

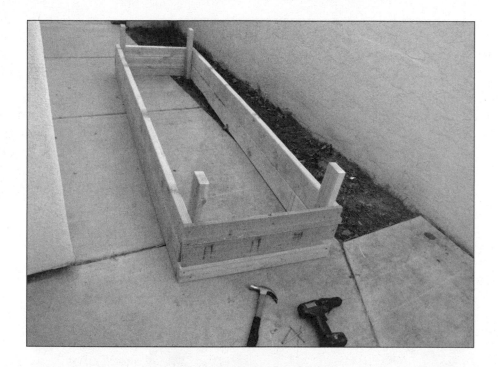

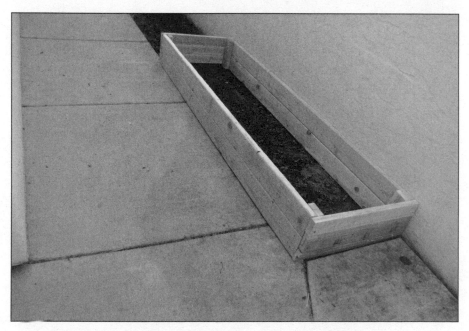

A raised bed built from old boards for an urban garden.

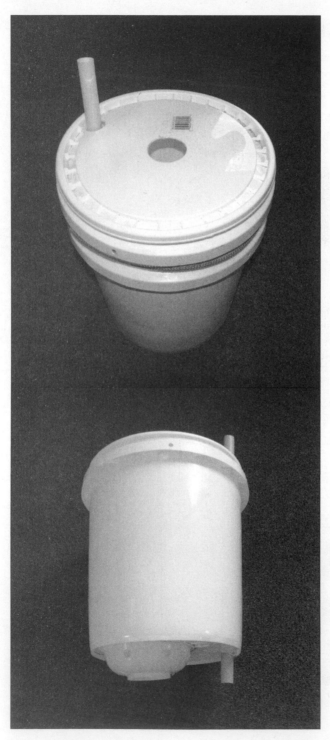

A self-watering five-gallon bucket planter is big enough for herbs or a medium-sized plant. This is made from two stacked five-gallon buckets. The inner bucket is modified as shown in the photo 5-3. A similar contraption made from large plastic storage tubs will hold a couple of tomato or half a dozen mature lettuce plants.

    i.   If you have some exposed soil, build it up with a raised bed, simple rock, or lumber walls a foot or two high to hold the soil.

    ii.   Containers can include commercial planting pots, stacked tires, kiddie pools, buckets, etc.

  d. Avoid tilling the soil.

  e. Rotate crops to prevent nutrient depletion and disease.

  f. Don't use pesticides or herbicides.

5. Watering

Coyne and Knutzen recommend watering deeply and less frequently. Use drip systems or soaker hose. Keep the soil spongy, not dripping wet, and let plants dry out slightly between watering.

6. Watch for infestations and diseases. Clip diseased foliage off and pick or wash off aphids or other damaging bugs.

7. Not all bugs and animal visitors are bad. Ladybugs, birds, spiders, and bees are good for a garden.

8. Consider concentrating on edible perennials (plants that come back year after year without replanting), such as fruit and nut trees. Dwarf varieties can be grown in large pots or buckets and will deliver plenty of fruit.

9. The key is to get started early. The garden needs to be already planted or at least ready to be planted if you expect to produce food when you need it. Just use the process and store the food you produce and keep the garden going. You can buy seedlings at any nursery in season and transplant them wherever you want, or you can store them and start your own seeds.

Some seeds start growing when planted per package directions directly in the ground. Others require special handling. Generally, here are the rules of thumb for starting seeds indoors:

1. Start a month before planting season.

2. Store seeds properly in a cool and dark location. (A refrigerator works well.)

3. Wide, flat containers prevent overcrowding. Plastic pots with good drainage are always the best to start with. Get some plant trays from the nursery, or drill some drainage holes in those old yogurt containers. Then all you have to do is add some potting soil.

4. Place seeds as directed on the soil and tamp the seeds with the bottom of a glass or bottle to ensure they make direct contact with the soil. Sprinkle some sphagnum moss or chicken grit to help keep the surface dry (helps prevent plant infections).

5. You can prevent plant infections by providing ventilation (consider a small fan on the lowest setting) and good drainage.

6. Make sure that you never overwater. Maintain the moisture level by covering the pots with plastic wrap. Check for dryness daily, and if more moisture is needed, spritz the surface soil with a spray bottle or place the pot in another container of water just deep enough to allow water to wick into the pot. Remove the plastic wrap when the seeds germinate.

7. Keeping the plant at a normal room temperature (65–75°F) encourages germination.

8. Expose (indoors) to sunlight or artificial light twelve to sixteen hours each day. Rotate the pot a quarter turn daily in relation to the available light source.

9. A weak fertilizer solution can be used once to encourage growth when the true leaves have appeared. The earliest leaves will probably be rounded food storage cells. True leaves resemble their adult versions.

10. Acclimate seedlings to direct sunlight temperature changes by exposing them outside for increasing periods over several days to prepare them for transplantation.

Some seeds require even more preparation, and there will usually be instructions to that effect on the seed package.

Many urban gardening manuals recommend growing only foods that are normally scarce or expensive. But the goal of a retreat, in contrast to convenience or savings, is sustainability. You're not only going to want the small scarce or expensive stuff like berries and herbs, instead you'll want to be able to produce the inexpensive staples like potatoes, onions, corn, squash, peppers, lettuce, carrots, tomatoes, beets, garlic, etc.

The following websites are excellent sources of information on how to grow and stores these types of foods:

www.gardeners.com/how-to/storing-potatoes-onions-garlic-squash/5021.html

www.gardenguides.com/114522-make-own-seed-potatoes .html

www.garden.org/learn/library/foodguide/veggie/#cat301

www.gardenguides.com/130505-corn-seed-spacing-planting-depth.html

www.thespruce.com/container-gardening-tips-4127751

MEAT AND DAIRY SUPPLEMENTATION

It's possible, of course, to surround a large, remote retreat with cattle and other animals for meat, eggs, and milk. But when the zombie hordes attack and the residents are forced to withdraw to the confines of their defensive perimeter, they will suddenly be forced to make do with not much more farming and ranching space than a typical urban or suburban retreat. This brief description of supplemental sources of meat and eggs applies to remote retreats as much as it does to urban ones.

When you take on this task, you will have to learn some important skills:

- How to slaughter, skin, and butcher your own meat.

- How to prevent attacks by common wild predators, like coyotes, foxes, skunks, raccoons, and even domestic pets by using fencing and other strategies.
- How to store meat and eggs so that they last and don't rot.
- What animals need for food, water, shelter, tolerance to weather, and temperature extremes.
- How to supplement your food with animal products, and to supplement their food with your scraps and fields.
- The basics of animal health and first aid.

There are many choices of animals to raise on small-scale farms, including the following:

1. Chickens

Chickens are a favored source of meat, eggs, and fertilizer. They are easy to care for and only need to be kept in a pen or small yard. Chickens, turkeys, ducks, and geese can forage for weeds and bugs (insects, snails, worms) in a field or pasture or even your container garden when it's not in season, which is important to sustaining a successful farm. Their waste can be tossed in the composter to speed up decomposition. They can fly over fences and are considered tasty by predators, so it's best to clip their wings to avoid that; and they must, of course, be well-watered and properly fed. Chickens are allowed in most rural and suburban areas, even if they're just kept as pets. In most suburban and urban areas, there's likely to be a ban on roosters due to the fact that they can make a lot of noise. Turkeys tend to roam a bit, but chickens tend to stay close to home, and if they do roam, will return home for the evening.

Chicken FAQs:

- Where do I get chickens?
  Get them as chicks from the local feed store. Make sure you know the sex so that you get all hens and no roosters.

- Do I need a rooster?
  No, hens will lay unfertilized eggs without a rooster present. If you want to breed chickens, you'll need a rooster.

- What breed and size are good for eggs?
  Leghorns, Rhode Island Reds, and Plymouth Rocks are good layers. Bantams are small but still lay a decent-size egg.

- What's the life expectancy of a laying hen?
  Three to eight years. Most hens can start laying at twenty weeks old and stop laying eggs at about the age of three.

- How many hens will I need?
  In a rural area, you can keep as many as you can handle. For an urban setting, three to five will keep a family of two in eggs every day (about a dozen per week).

- Is raising them for meat practical?
  Raising chickens or ducks for meat is quite time consuming and very costly. Wait until a hen stops laying then cook it up.

- What do I do with the starter chicks?
  Keep them warm, hydrated, and fed. A cardboard box heated with a 60-watt lamp bulb makes an adequate "brooder."

- What is a henhouse?
  This is a box with roosting bars and a few nesting boxes. It's where they sleep and lay eggs. The house and the fenced "run" that surrounds it are what we call a coop.

- What should I feed them?
  For your chicks, most feed stores sell a special type of chick feed that works well. Adults like scratch (cracked grains), greens, vegetable scraps, and fruit. They need grit, either from the dirt or store-bought. They also use a lot of calcium, so you can boil egg shells and feed it to them to supply the vitamins they need.

- Some good chicken websites?
  www.backyardchickens.com/articles/how-to-raise-chickens.47660
  en.wikibooks.org/wiki/Raising_Chickens
  web.archive.org/web/20161030130509/http://www.mybackyardchickenfarm.com/index.html
  web.archive.org/web/20170708195604/http://www.lionsgrip.com/chickens.html
  poultry.ces.ncsu.edu/small-flock-management-resources

2. Ducks
   Ducks are a little noisier than chickens but are a good source of meat and eggs and they eat plenty of garden bugs.

Duck FAQs:

- Where do I get ducks?
  You can get them at the same feed store as you would get chicks.

- Do I need a drake (male)?
  No, unless you plan to raise ducks.

- What breeds are good layers?

Most often recommended is the Khaki Campbell. Indian Runners are better layers but have other issues that put them in second place.

- How many do I need?
  At least two, as ducks get lonely.

- How do I handle the chicks?
  The same way you would with chickens, by using a brooder box.

- Do I need a duck coop (house + run)?
  Yes, but no brooding bars are needed.

- What do ducks eat?
  Plants (including weeds and garden plants), bugs, and duck feed.

- Will they need a swimming pond?
  Ducks use deep water to drink and clean themselves. A kiddie pool will do, but change the water daily. (Best idea is to use it in the garden.)

  A great duck site:
  duckhobby.com

3. Geese
These birds are noisy and aggressive but are an excellent source of meat and eggs and feathers/down. Ducks and geese like the water, which gives you another reason to raise fish. A great goose site:
www.motherearthnews.com/homesteading-and-livestock/raising-ducks-geese/keeping-geese-ze0z10zhir

4. Turkeys

Turkeys are most often raised for meat, and a single bird can provide fifty pounds of it. Turkeys are not prolific egg layers, and most spoiled Americans who try turkey eggs are not particularly fond of them. Here are a couple of good websites:

poultry.ces.ncsu.edu/small-flock-management-resources
www.frugal-living-freedom.com/raising-turkeys.html

5. Quail, Pheasant, Pigeon

Quail are comparatively small but are reliable and frequent layers. The chicks mature in about six weeks or so, creating lots of eggs and meat in a short amount of time. Pigeons are also easy to raise and reproduce quickly, though, as with guinea pigs, most Americans have a difficult time with the idea of eating one. Both quail and pigeons fly, so they're often clipped or kept in barns or coops. Breeding pheasants is much like breeding chickens.

These are good game bird sites:

web.archive.org/web/20140220123748/http://www.ehow.com:80/how_5682938_raise-wild-game-birds.html
www.wikihow.com/Breed-Quail

6. Rabbits

Rabbits require little room and provide meat, fur, and fertilizer. They're very quiet and can be kept in small pens. You can also let them roam around in the grass, but they'll require herding home at the end of the day. Rabbits will eat anything green, and their waste is excellent in a composter or, after it has dried as a fertilizer. A male and a couple of females can act as breeders and multiply "like rabbits." A single doe can produce as much as 1,000 times her own weight in meat per year. The common meat breeds are New Zealand's and Californians, but Angora rabbits are a good choice, since they can provide meat and fertilizer and their long hair can be combed out when they molt and spun into yarn.

Some great rabbit sites:
web.archive.org/web/20100829104355/http://www.thefarm.org:80/charities/i4at/lib2/rabbits.htm
www.essortment.com/raising-meat-rabbits-41673.html

7. Guinea Pigs
Female guinea pigs can have five litters a year of one to six babies, and the females of the litter can have their own pups just a month after birth. Again, two females and a male will keep you in meat. They are very cheap to feed and the meat is high in protein and low in fat and cholesterol. Raising guinea pigs is much like raising rabbits, just a bit noisier. A great guinea pig site:
ginneypig.com

8. Fish
Fish can be nearly self-sufficient with adequate water surface area and depth. Depending on the species, they do well in warm, cold, deep, shallow, or moving water. They can eat bugs, other fish, some plants, and some are straight bottom feeders.
Some sites:
www.motherearthnews.com/homesteading-and-livestock/backyard-fish-farming-zmaz06amzwar
www.hunker.com/13424254/how-to-raise-catfish-in-a-barrel
The second site above is a great site with a relatively easy method of raising fish in a 55-gallon barrel. Clean harvested water can be used. The project requires an aquarium filter which could be run on its own 5-watt solar cell and battery (<$80). The water must be changed daily, but is nutrient rich and can be used to water the garden.

9. Goats

Goats are the only animal on this list that provides both meat and milk. One assumes it would fairly easy to raise goats, but when your goats have babies, you'll run out of space and ground forage in a hurry. You'll need about fifteen square feet of barn space per adult. A three-sided shelter is enough, but it will need to be secured with a stout woven-wire fence at least four feet high. A large chain link commercial kennel is an excellent alternative. Any goat can provide meat, but not all are excellent milk producers. Nubian goats seem to be the most often recommended dairy goats. Goats will eat almost anything vegetable, including weeds, leaves, grass, and scraps or discards from the kitchen and garden. Dairy goats should be fed a daily chunk of alfalfa hay if it's available.

A few goat sites:

If you've got lots of space, visit this one…

http://animals.mom.me/how-to-start-a-goat-farm-4938376.html

If you live in the city, try this one:

www.mnn.com/your-home/organic-farming-gardening/stories/how-to-keeping-goats-city

10. Bees

These are silent and clean creatures that can be safely kept on a rooftop, balcony, or unenclosed patio. One hive can easily supply more honey than a small family can use.

Bee Basics:

- A simple bee kit with hive, frames, smoker, personal protective gear, gadgets and tools, and instructions can be had for as little as $160.
- A three-pound package of 10,000 bees with a queen will probably cost at least $100 plus delivery. The other option is to bring home wild bees.
- The queen bee lives about two or three years. Worker bees work themselves to death in four to six weeks during the late spring and summer but live much longer in winter.

- It will take months for the bees to do their work, so like everything else we've discussed in this book, you've got to get started before TSHTF.
- Bees attack to protect the honey and young. They are far more sedated when they're swarming because they are away from the hive.
- Before you go through all the expense, check with neighbors and local codes, as not everyone likes the idea of bees next door. Tell neighbors you'll slip them some honey when it's ready and explain to them that you will place the hive where the bee flight paths do not intersect with human traffic.

www.chelseagreen.com/blogs/urban-apiculture-or-bees-in-the-city-draft

http://outdoorplace.org/beekeeping/citybees.htm

Check out these sites to learn how to harvest honey:

web.archive.org/web/20110912024357/gomestic.com/gardening/harvesting-honey-from-bee-hives

web.archive.org/web/20100505065044/www.ehow.com/how_1649_harvest-honey.html

The following website is a great source of information on animal farming:

www.frugal-living-freedom.com

WATER SUSTAINABILITY

If you've got property for a rural retreat, it may be possible to drill a well or find and prepare a spring. Refer to *Living off the Grid* for additional information and references to well and spring resources.

WATER HARVESTING

If a well or spring is not available, the answer to water sustainability is conservation and the art of catchment systems, or water harvesting. A water catchment system works where wells can't be dug, groundwater is contaminated, springs can't be found, or rain is scarce. These types of systems have been used for thousands of years in countries with poor groundwater resources. Even in the desert, a short rain can deliver enough water to keep the household going until the next storm.

The easiest form of storm harvesting is a simple rain barrel fed by the downspout of the rain gutters or edges of a building. Yes, the water will certainly be dirty, but metal or clay tile roofs seem to be cleaner than shingled roofs. For a little extra, there are many commercial rain barrels available with perks like roof-cleaner diverters and prebarrel filters.

Water from a barrel is not pressurized, except by gravity, but that gives it just enough pressure to water a garden using a hose from the barrel drain. Elevating the barrel, using cinder blocks, increases the pressure, but it won't support a plumbing system of any kind without a pump. Storm-harvesting systems intended to provide water for drinking, cooking, and bathing will need pumping, filtration, and disinfection systems.

The harvesting system may also drain into larger above-ground tanks, underground cisterns, or into dammed reservoirs. Some commercial versions also have roof-cleaning diverters.

Aside from roofs, melt- and rainwater can be captured from gullies and washes, but the obvious problem is sediment (mud) buildup and the control of raging floodwaters. Large systems like this can become hazards to anything downstream.

Some old-school methods are a little more labor-intensive but happen to work quite well. Excavate the available land area so impermeable surfaces (cement, pavement, etc.) are minimized and the ground is morphed in a way that it catches the rain and funnels it in the direction you want it to go as irrigation or catch-water. Terracing is a simple method of keeping rain- and melt-water from running away. Directing the water into a mulch basin is another effective variation. Mulch basins are pits or trenches planted with high crops (large plants or trees) and covered with mulch. A mulch basin is also a good place to send gray water if the basin has been planted with alkaline-tolerant plants. Try this website for ideas: www.thegardenhelper.com/alkalineplants.html

A cistern is a tank made of concrete, steel, fiberglass, or plastic and can sit either above- or belowground. If the cistern or water tank is aboveground and higher than the building's internal plumbing, the weight of the water in the cistern may provide adequate pressure. Otherwise, a pump is needed to send water from the catchment to the house. Again, filtering and disinfection will be needed before using the water for drinking, cooking, or bathing. A rain barrel or any other aboveground storage device requires steps to keep it from freezing.

GREYWATER

Domestic wastewater is made up of greywater and blackwater. Greywater comes from the laundry, bathroom sink, shower or tub, kitchen, and various appliances. Basically, it's any wastewater that's not contaminated with feces. Blackwater comes from the toilet and is usually referred to as sewage. Blackwater is highly infectious, but it's not the same for greywater. While blackwater must be purified and treated before it can be reused, greywater, which also carries germs and pollutants, can be reused to water gardens. As a rule of thumb, don't use greywater on crops that anyone might eat raw, and don't let it sit around in barrels or ponds as it will soon turn foul.

Since most of your greywater is going to come from the shower, sink, and washing machine, it's a good idea to try to control the pollutants by using greywater-friendly detergents. The information on the bottle or box should specifically say whether it's greywater friendly or not. Common detergents have chemical additives that make them incompatible with greywater systems.

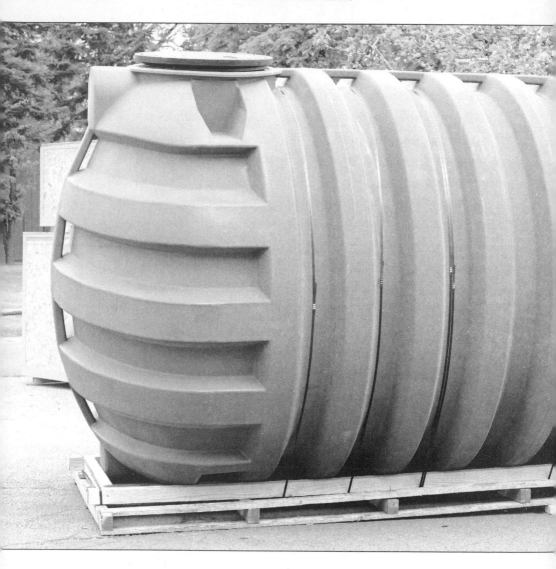

Greywater systems range from simple and inexpensive to highly complex and very expensive. All greywater systems rely on two principles: the first being that healthy topsoil can purify or filter greywater, and the second is that humans cannot use greywater for watering crops, drinking, cooking, or bathing before it is purified.

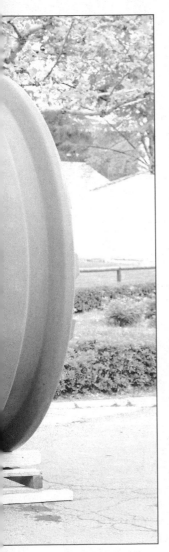

The simplest method of reusing greywater is to just drain it or dump it in buckets directly onto garden soil. Use a bucket to collect any water that has to run to heat up. After a bath or during a shower, remember to siphon water to the bucket or to an outside location. It takes little effort to disconnect the pipes under the sink, so drainage will go into a large bucket or to add a pipe or hose that will carry it directly outside where it's needed. Sophisticated systems treat gray water prior to disposal by using in-line filters or settling tanks and sand filters in order to remove pollutants and germs before distributing it through a drip system.

Keep in mind that greywater tinged with detergents is going to be alkalized. Make sure you do not direct that kind of water to plants that you know are not alkali-resistant. There are several lists of alkali-resistant plants on the Internet. Use your search engine to pull them up. A better idea is to use detergent-contaminated gray water for other purposes, like flushing toilets.

A greywater system is based on site, climate, budget, quantity, need of soil permeability, how much work you're willing to do, and local health and building codes. Once you go beyond the basic methods mentioned above, you'll need a working knowledge of basic plumbing and the tools to accomplish it. The Internet is rifled with DIY information and tutorials. Again, we'll recommend the book *The Urban Homestead* for a great introduction to inexpensive alternatives.

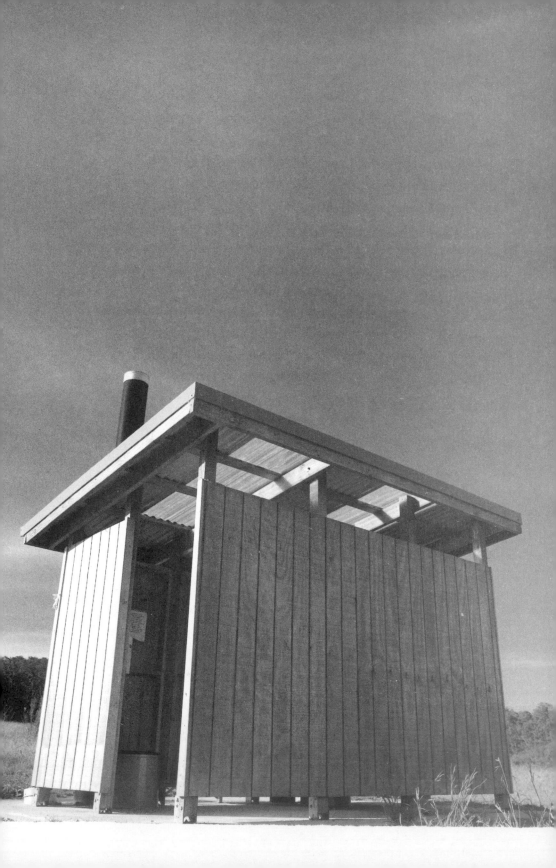

For most people, greywater is easiest to handle within a septic system. Separate black- and greywater systems are easy to install during new construction, but to modify an existing dwelling to handle separate systems is difficult and very expensive.

Let's pause briefly for a return to reality. In a true "shit hits the fan" scenario, you're not going to have the luxury of a public water utility, and you'll be wishing that you had a spring or a well. You're going to be using water you've stored and whatever water you have been able to harvest. Conservation will be king as there will be no room for wasting any water—clean or grey.

DEALING WITH HUMAN WASTE

While rural retreats in worst-case scenarios are still going to have functional septic systems, urban and suburban retreaters are likely to be on public sewer systems, which will eventually fail and back up. Retreat builders would be wise to invest in composting toilets. Commercial systems come in all shapes and sizes, from septic systemlike basement chambers to individual toilets that must be emptied into other containers. A DIY version is a simple five-gallon bucket, with or without a toilet seat modified to fit it. Cover each "extraction" with a carbonaceous material (sawdust) or even sand to reduce the odor. If you've got a big supply of buckets, just fill the bucket, seal it with the lid, and store where it won't become an aesthetic or health risk. If you've just got one or two buckets, then line them with a couple of strong garbage bags. When the bucket is nearly full, pull the bags out and seal them. Double bagging is important, but of course, if the situation is prolonged, the bags and the buckets will run out. Even then, there are solutions. Some advice:

humanurehandbook.com

www.relianceproducts.com/products/sanitation.html

Chapter 6

A Closer Look at Defense and Security

DEFENSE STRATEGY 101

DON'T GIVE THE ZOMBIES THE INFORMATION THEY NEED TO MAKE IT *attractive or easy.*

A planned act of aggression against a target is based on information (intelligence) about the target. Deliberate misinformation or denial of information is a huge component of security. Remember to always keep a low profile and don't share your plans or inventories with strangers or those that you do not 100 percent trust. Occasionally, change or alter your lifestyle patterns (what time you leave the home, what route you take, which vehicle you use, which door to the house you favor)

Use a combination of passive (soft) and active (hard) defense methods.

Passive defense methods are those which impose the perception of insignificance, inconvenience, danger, complications, and the need for exaggerated effort. They are aimed at making a target less important than it is, largely by denying access. For passive methods, invisibility is the first level or layer of protection. This means that you must be covert and incognito. This does not mean having to move to a desert in Southern Idaho, just don't make yourself a target; camouflage or otherwise blend into the natural or urban surroundings. Appear as if you have no more than the average household or that it would be dangerous or inconvenient to mess with you. Do this in a way that does not imply a well-stocked cache of goodies. Avoid signs that imply that you're well equipped, but provide a perceptibly inhospitable reception.

Consider announcing reasons to stay away. In rural areas, try signs that imply radioactive, chemical, or infectious contamination or other thought-provoking threats as opposed to signs that imply the presence of "booty" (High Voltage, Protected by xxxxx Security, Guard Dog on Duty, KEEP OUT, Private Property, No Trespassing, Video Surveillance).

If your goal is to be rural and remote, then cover your tracks. Create natural obstacles that don't imply major importance (trees and rocks rather than new barbed wire, high fences, and cement). Remove indicators of civilization (tracks, noise, machinery, vehicles, noisy radios, generators, smoke plumes, lights at night, working chimneys, visible gardens, vehicle parks, fresh refuse, laundry hanging on a line, mowed lawns, and tended yards).

Most suburban and urban retreaters will, of course, consider other preventive protection resources, including structural modifications (fences and other barriers, exterior window and door reinforcements, etc.), electronics (alarm and monitor systems), and lifestyle changes, such as keeping pets (guard dogs). The visibility and pros and cons of these measures should be carefully thought out. Is the protection it affords greater than the attention it draws?

In addition to structural modifications, there's a seemingly endless list of passive measures that can include perimeter guards, listening and observation posts, antivehicular ditches (for the super paranoid), and concertina wire obstacles. Security spikes can be installed on walls, fences, gates, and roofs. Glass shards from broken bottles—the poor man's spikes—can be cemented in place where needed.

To prevent intruders from climbing to attain access to upper levels, low tree limbs or nearby trees can be cut down or cut back. Thorny bushes or cacti can be planted at the base of a wall (rosebushes, prickly pear, yucca, barberry, hawthorn, holly, firethorn, bramble, locust, rose).

Another issue often addressed by survivalist die-hards is night combat, and the point is well taken. Intruders cannot negotiate your structure's territory in the dark like you can. Appropriate tactics may include having exterior lights to observe the perimeter or no lights on in the house at night and, when leaving the structure at night, leaving a light on inside the structure to enable you to see silhouettes inside when you return.

Fencing can provide a degree of passive defense as long as it does not also provide cover for intruders. Stout barbed wire fencing and chain link are examples of perimeter fencing that keep the intruder visible and exposed.

Active methods are aggressively physical methods ranging from running away to a full-combat response. A lot of what is considered passive defense (certain structural modifications) are platforms for an active response. Popular and influential survivalist writers Jeff Cooper and James Wesley Rawles are proponents of an aggressive style of defense focusing on firearms and exterior perimeter security. Cooper, in his book, *Notes on Tactical Residential Architecture*, touts the Vauban principle—that one or more projecting corner bastions permit observation of multiple walls and the perimeter, allowing easier defense against flanking maneuvers. This is best done as the structure is built, starting at the blueprint design; but adding a bastion or two on corners of a preexisting structure is not an unreasonable task if the funds are available. One bastion will be able to cover two walls, and two will be able to cover all four walls of a squared structure. Occasionally, a structure will be backed on one wall or more by a cliff or may be built into a hillside, precluding the need for coverage on that side.

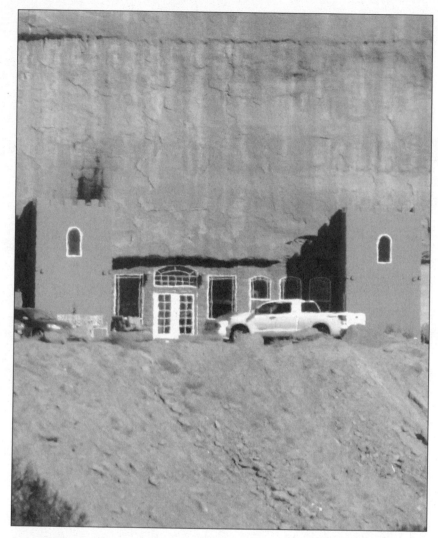

An attack on this retreat can come from only one direction. The towers provide 180-degree cover from above. Attempts by intruders to gain entry would be easily controlled with firepower from the two sides.

European-style courtyard designs, with open space surrounded by the home, and a long narrow entryway with hardened exterior walls are options for funneling intruders into an entryway ambush. For the super paranoid, there are even more threatening defensive devices. (Like fougasses, the common man's IED—

ideally activated by a trip wire, made by filling hollows or tubes in the ground with explosives and projectiles and mantrap foyers (called a "crushroom" by Rawles), entryways that can be sprayed with bullets or toxic gases as an ambush. At a minimum, some insist that all entry doorways should be recessed in such a way that the house surrounds anyone at the door so they can be viewed from several angles, exposing the intruder from front, side, and back. This, of course, requires a port for viewing; and if you're planning to blast your visitor with gunfire, the port should be unscreened, narrow, and easily opened. Of course, any wall that contains an observation/firing port must be small arms-fireproof. Sheetrock is cosmetic and will not stop a bullet.

Keep it safe for the family.
In the rush to build a survivalist retreat, protect the family from the hazards they will be exposed to. For example, that high-voltage stun device under the carpet is just as likely to shock your kids as it is an intruder.

Be reasonable with your hard defense considerations. Weapons, especially firearms, can be a tremendous deterrent. They give the defender a dash of psychological security, and nobody, not even a zombie marauder, wants to get shot in the face. Of course, the option to arm may sooner or later disappear since private gun ownership is constantly under attack.

Die-hard survivalists insist on the necessity for the immediate availability of weaponry for a hard response. While going without weapons certainly causes no harm and eliminates the threats of family suicides and homicides with those weapons, the absence of such weapons in an EOTW bedlam situation would increase the likelihood of successful victimization. If you decide to arm your home or retreat, you *must* do the training to learn the skills to efficiently use the weapon. Hunting, target shooting, and safety classes are of little use. Combat (tactical and urban warfare) shooting skills are needed. Take a course from a combat shooting school that has instructors with real combat experience. There are now a couple of hundred thousand urban combat veterans in this country who would be far more qualified than the average safety range instructor. Find someone who speaks to the point, is easily understood, and who approaches things from a problem-solving angle rather than a "kill 'em all" mentality.

Follow state and federal regulations for purchasing the weapons and consider getting a concealed weapon permit even though you plan to keep your weapons at home or at the retreat. You have to get them from the store to your home to your retreat, and just moving them in a vehicle can get you arrested if the local gun laws are vague about concealment. When you've got them home, use trigger guards and gun safes to protect the family.

Once you've got the weapons and the skills, they key is to practice, practice, practice. Don't forget to have adequate ammunition on hand. Recommendations vary enormously depending on the "expert," but a couple of hundred rounds for carbines and handguns and fifty or so for shotguns would be a rational minimum.

Recognize the potential threats and develop practical actions and procedures to deal with them.
A popular mnemonic *see it through* is often used to help remember a simple procedure for dealing with threats. Survey, evaluate, execute. Several modern survivalist writers propose learning and using military-style tactical thinking in which incoming information is constantly used to redefine the situation and modify the response. OODA (Boyd's Cycle) is big among survivalists. Have any questions, just Google it.

Know your territory.
Think about how you and intruders will maneuver and where the likely points of entry are. How will you know when or where

there's been a breach? Do you have alarms and observation equipment? Is there enough cover for you and yours but limited cover for attackers in those last ten yards or so leading to your location? Do you know the topography of your area, and in urban areas can you envision the buildup as terrain (buildings as high points, basements and sewers as caves, alleyways and hallways as canyons and tunnels?).

There is safety in numbers.
In urban and suburban scenarios, consider planning with neighbors. A neighborhood with a lot of security and firepower, where intruders check in but don't check out, will be avoided by the zombie hordes.

When the last lines of defense are being threatened, shift into MacGyver mode.
Suggestions for prefortifying the structure are given throughout this book. If you haven't taken these precautions, in an emergency, nonessential windows could be boarded up with plywood. Remember, though, that most walls are made with Sheetrock. Nailing a plywood sheet to Sheetrock is futile unless the nails or screws go into the struts behind them.

Employ distractions and deception as needed. Here is where your close-range weapons will come into play. Those weapons can include tasers, baseball bats, pepper spray, pistols, and shotguns.

If you intend to actively defend your site, know the basics of combat. Popular survivalist writers recommend some simple ideas:

a) Understand the reality of your situation. Defenders are essentially stuck in a fixed position, but attackers are mobile. They can flank, siege, pin, snipe infiltrate, or charge. Talk to urban combat veterans for some basic tips. Identify your overall strategy and know your place in it.

b) Retreat is not a dirty word. Retreating disrupts the attacker's tactics and forces him to him to rethink. But you must have somewhere to retreat to. Unless you've planned your retreat with an escape route or a safe room, you won't have that option. Develop a plan to evacuate and predetermine a location and a time to rally.

c) Consider a counterattack. The enemy will be surprised and may be caught without defensive fortifications.

d) Ambushes are devastating but require good intelligence, cover, and concealment.

e) Use cross fire whenever possible. This is the idea behind Vauban bastions by making the attacker defend against two or more positions/directions.

f) Be realistic in your approach. Fighting off the zombie hordes is one thing, defending against a full military assault is another. If you become the object of a military offensive, it's all over. You may delay a few tanks, APC's, or Strykers with old antitank tactics, but you cannot hope to successfully defend yourself against a modern organized army with today's "smart weaponry" (satellite surveillance, offensive drone weapons, satellite- and laser-guided precision bombs and missiles, and weapons like the MOAB, a bunker-busting mega bomb called the Mother of All Bombs). Resistance against a modern government-backed military machine is futile.

DEFENSIVE FIREARMS

Of all the topics in the survivalism realm, armament is by far the most controversial. The mere possession of a firearm in the home enormously increases the likelihood that you or a loved one will be killed by it. While I have spent much my life with weapons in

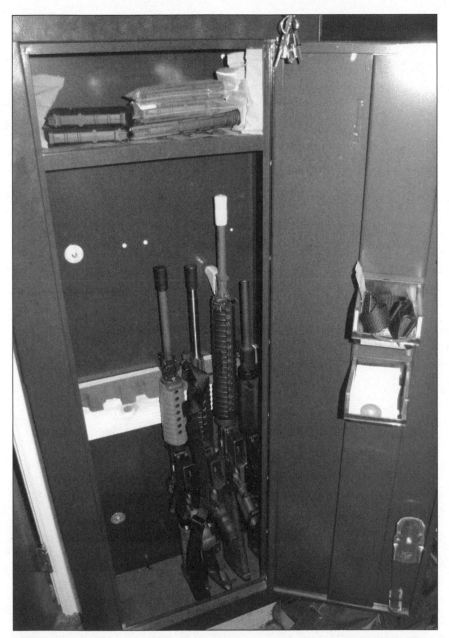

This gun safe is one of two used to store ammunition and a dozen rifles and handguns in the basement of a small urban retreat in Northern Utah. The owner keeps his first choice of firepower, a Mossberg 590 12–gauge shotgun with a hundred rounds of 00 buckshot, locked in the ground-floor hall closet.

the home and did twelve years in the military, in my seven years as a paramedic in the American West, I encountered hundreds of gunshot wounds, and by far, the majority of them were suicides. The rest were accidents or resulted from domestic disputes. None of them were defensive in nature, a fact which pretty much verifies the statistics the gun-control crowd is using. In spite of that, there won't be any preaching in this book.

With that said, it is only ethical to tell the readers that if they can spend a couple of thousand dollars on an arms cache, they can certainly spend a couple hundred to protect their family from the additional hazard. Unless there's an imminent danger of attack, guns should be stored, unloaded, with trigger locks in place. Ammunition should be stored and locked up separately. A more convenient solution is a gun safe secured to the floor or wall studs. A five-gun safe can be had for $150. A package of four trigger locks costs about $10. They're cheap insurance.

Here are some simple, basic firearms guidelines:
1. Know the firearms laws of your country, state, county, and city. Search your own conscience. Decide before an incident just what constitutes a reasonable, legitimate reason to kill another person.
2. Keep your weapon clean.
3. Always open and check the chamber and magazine when you pick up a firearm.
4. Never point a gun at someone you're not intending to shoot.
5. Be aware of your backdrop. Anything behind the target is in danger of getting hit, even if it's in the other room. Walls don't stop bullets. Overpenetration can be reduced by careful selection of caliber and ammunition.

6. Keep your finger off the trigger until you're ready to shoot.
7. Choose a firearm capable of stopping the threat. Ask yourself: Is the caliber substantial enough? Can I aim it correctly? Will it hold enough ammunition to do the job?
8. Choose a reliable firearm, one that doesn't have a history of jamming or malfunctioning. Check consumer reports on the Internet for this information.
9. Shop around. You don't need to go broke or starve your children to get your firearms. There are some good inexpensive firearms available.

SHOTGUNS

A 12-gauge pump-action shotgun and large-gauge buckshot rounds are by far the firearm and ammo most recommended by experts, including gun shop owners, for home defense. There are several reasons for this. When fired, they spread those big buckshot pellets over a wider area than a bullet, giving them tremendous stopping power. The rounds are also easy to find and relatively inexpensive—as little as forty cents each. Their design is simple, and malfunctions are very rare.

Gauge refers to the diameter of the barrel or the shell. The most preferred shell is often the 12-gauge 2¾ inch. It's the most common and easiest to find. Shotgun shells are filled with pellets or fragments. "Double-ought" shot gives a good spread. Because a 12g 2¾ inch double-ought shell contains seven to nine pellets just slightly smaller than the diameter of a 9mm bullet, a single shot can be nearly as effective as firing a full clip of pistol rounds. The range is good too. Even at fifty yards, a well-aimed 12g shotgun is still a formidable deterrent.

There's enough power in a 12g that the possibility of shooting through the wall and hitting family members has to be

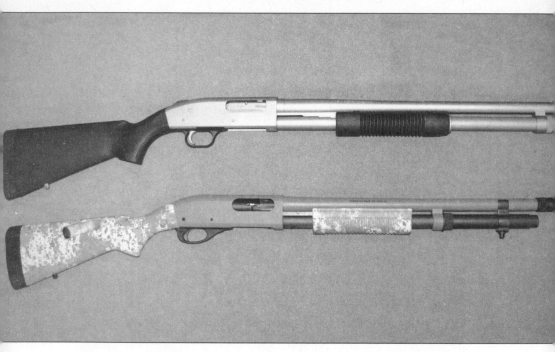

A Mossberg 590 (top) and a Remington 870 tactical shotgun (bottom). The 870 has long been an icon for home defense and at the time of this writing runs about $300 for the basic model. Interstate Arms makes a tactical model similar to the 870 (the CIA Ultra 87) that sells at $185.

considered. To mitigate overpenetration, some survivalists have recommended no. 1 (ten .30mm pellets) or smaller buckshot, or no. 4–6 Birdshot, which has more pellets (130 or so), more spread, less chance of going through the wall, and less recoil but sacrifices substantial stopping power.

Classic Home Defenders: Mossberg 500, Mossberg Maverick 88, Remington 870 (18-inch barrel).
Budget Alternatives: Interstate Arms Defender, Hi Point CIA Ultra 87.

The 12g shotguns kick like a mule, and after a few rounds, your shoulder will be destroyed for the day. Talk to your trainer or gun dealer about ways to reduce the effects of the recoil. Ammunition capacity (usually four to eight rounds) is another disadvantage of shotguns, but their spread and stopping power make up for it.

Don't fall prey to the myth that you don't need to aim a shotgun. At twenty-five feet, the spread averages eight inches, but at 120 feet, the spread is going to be five feet with only 40 percent (or three to four) of the pellets hitting within a 30-inch bull's-eye. This means you could completely miss the target if your aim is a degree or two off. Practice frequently and learn how to aim your shotgun. Filing the sights off a BB gun and using it to practice is a cheap and effective way of learning how to aim a shotgun without bruising your shoulder.

HANDGUNS

Survivalists generally go for semiautomatic handguns using magazines rather than revolvers. The three most common calibers are 9mm, .40 cal., and .45 cal. While .40s and .45s have greater stopping power, there are certainly advantages to choosing a 9mm

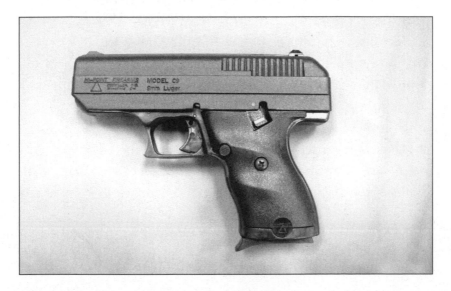

A good low-cost alternative is the Hi-Point C9 Comp (9mm), running at $130–160.

weapon. Less recoil means being better able to keep on target. Smaller caliber means increased capacity of magazines and a lighter weapon. Plus, 9mm is now the most common handgun ammunition, not including .22.

Another advantage of choosing a 9mm handgun is that there are currently semiautomatic carbines (rifles) available that use 9mm pistol ammunition, giving the possibility of having two different home defense weapons that use the same inexpensive round. A Hi-Point combination, the C9 9mm compact pistol ($140 at Impact Arms) and the 9mm carbine ($225 at Cabellas) are inexpensive examples.

Ammunition: Most handguns hold seven to fifteen rounds. A hollow point round is generally recommended for home defense. It has plenty of stopping power, and because it spreads out, it has less chance of overpenetration in the home than a "ball" or FMJ (full metal jacket).

Most commonly recommended handguns: Modern polymer guns are popular today due to their light weight, lower cost, easy maintenance, and tough materials. Full-size handguns that are often recommended are the Springfield XD, Glock 17, Smith & Wesson M&P (9mm, .40, or .45 cal.) &, and the FN Herstal FNP 40 (.40 cal.). Popular concealable include the Glock 19 (9mm), the Glock 23 (.40 cal.), and the Glock 26 (9mm "Baby Glock").

Note that handguns are comparatively ineffective firearms. Their advantages have more to do with low cost, easy concealment, minimal malfunction, and easy storage than with effectiveness.

RIFLES

Unless hunting is part of your self-sustainment plan, or picking off intruders as they cross the open spaces between your picket fence and your front door is how you envision defending your

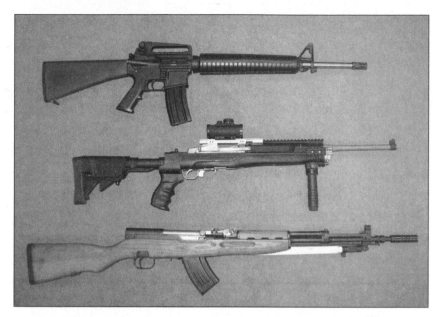

Local pawnshop booty (top to bottom): AR-15, Ruger Mini-14, SKS.

retreat, there's really not much reason to get a rifle. A pistol or a shotgun will do the trick. Some people, though, just want to have the extra accuracy, range, and effectiveness or want to be able to hunt game. Frangible rifle rounds are extremely lethal and rifles have greater accuracy and range than shotguns or handguns.

In survivalist circles, rifles are commonly limited to assault-type weapons. Like the psychology of the chick-chick of a pump shotgun, the romantic silhouettes of the AK-47 and M-16 (AR-15) draw retreaters to assault-style rifles like ants to sugar.

The most commonly purchased rifles for home defense and retreats are the AK-47 variants and SKSs because they are easily maintained. The AK-47 is the most common rifle in the world, and its 7.62 caliber is the most common rifle ammunition world-wide. Also popular are the AR-15 (M-16) variants and the Ruger "ranch rifles," the Mini-14 and the Mini-30. Generally speaking, you won't find any of these weapons new for under $350.

Ammunition: One of the advantages of these rifles is their high ammunition capacity. Clips that hold thirty-plus rounds are quite common. The most common rifle rounds in order of availability are the 7.62 x 39mm, used with most SKSs, AK-47s, and the Mini-30, the .223 (5.56mm) caliber Remington, used in the AR-15 and Mini-14, and the 5.62 x 45mm NATO round, also used in the AR-15 and Mini-14. Some weapons can use both the 5.62 and the .223. The cheapest of these rounds is the 7.62 x 39mm, available in hollow point, FMJ, and soft point.

Again, overpenetration is a big concern with these powerful weapons. "Frangible" ammunition can mitigate this to some degree. These rounds flatten and fragment when they hit something, which reduces penetration. Avoid using FMJ (full metal jacket) or HP (hollow point) ammunition within the confines of the retreat or home.

Budget Alternatives: the Hi-Point 9mm carbine.

Accessories: There are plenty of accessories available for your rifle. Larger-capacity clips, telescopic sights, laser sights, specialized stocks, tripods, flash suppressors, etc. If you've got the money, the shops have the toys.

Thinking about a .22 caliber sniper rifle? The Ruger 10/22 is an example of a small-caliber weapon that has enjoyed success as a sniper rifle. It was employed by the Israeli Army in Palestine and Gaza with good success. The .22LR (long rifle) ammunition is very cheap and available everywhere in the USA. The .22 rifle has virtually no recoil, and most are easily maintained. They are one of the more accurate rifles. A basic Ruger 10/22 costs between $200 and $500, depending on the model. An infinite supply of accessories is available, including twenty-five-round clips, high-tech scopes and sights, and tactical stocks. For a suppressed (silenced) version, expect to pay around a thousand dollars.

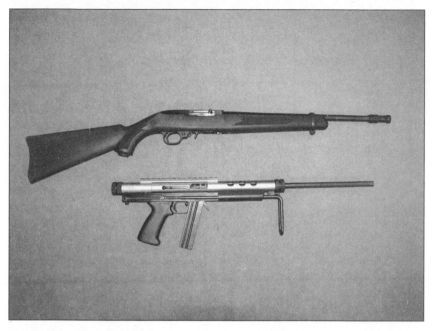

Top, a Ruger 10/22. Bottom, a FeatherUSA RAV-22 breakdown .22 caliber rifle.

By the way, the only retreat defense weapon it makes sense to silence, or suppress, is a rifle. Readers can find a great discussion on suppressors and silencers at

www.gun-shots.net/firearm-gun-silencers-suppressors.shtml

Chapter 7

Visits to Real Retreats

PRIVATE – An Urban Retreat Makeover

IN RESEARCHING THIS PROJECT, I SELECTED WHAT I CONSIDERED TO be an average apartment in an average urban neighborhood, rented by a middle-aged couple we'll call the Hahn family, with an average household income ($45,000 to 50,000 per year before taxes) and an average household debt ($18,000–20,000 not including rent). After bills, $1,000 monthly rent, and taxes, this average couple manages to have about a thousand per month left to pay utilities, insurance, buy food and prescriptions, handle transportation costs, pay for the kids' college, and manage miscellaneous expenses. Needless to say at this point, survival is an everyday concern for this family, not some Hollywood-fueled fear of alien space invasions or end-times doomsday diseases. Buying up a dandy parcel of prime wilderness to build their dream retreat is out of the question. But that shouldn't, and doesn't, exclude them from making preparations and modifications that can prepare them for even worse-case scenarios.

After squeezing the financial sponge for every drop, Dale and Crystal Hahn decided they could afford up to $2,000 over a period of twelve months, about $167 per month, to turn their home into a functional, reasonably self-sustaining retreat.

The residence structure was a single-story two-bed, two-bath triplex unit with a gated entry into a tiny patio where the main door is located. The triplex is one of many similar triplexes, forty units along both sides of a street a block long. Tight quarters, and it would be difficult imagining a viable retreat in this situation. To make things worse, the homeowners association rules with an iron fist and does not allow any modifications that would make any one of the units visually distinct from the others. Also, the aspect and shape of the structure limit exposure to the sun that might be used for solar energy collection or agriculture. To utilize the sun, the solar array would need to be mobile and moved from sunny spot to sunny spot during the day. Due to the extensive concrete coverage, there is also very limited access to open soil for farming (twenty-four square feet located inside the entry courtyard).

A good way to get started is to map out the entire house and grounds. Take notes on the likely threats and how they can be mitigated. Then prioritize.

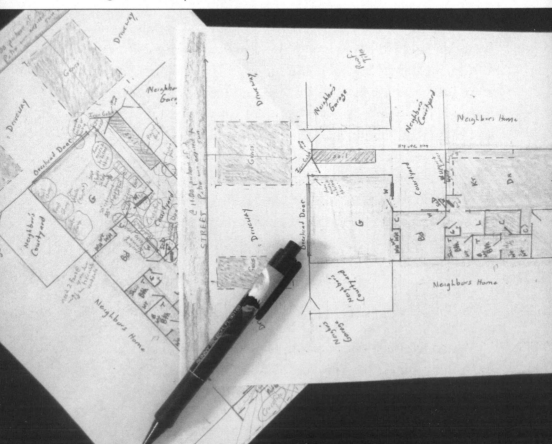

The Hahns started this project with a basic "dirty dozen" of tools. Eventually, they added a couple of items to that dozen, but for convenience, not necessity. The dirty dozen included a:

1. claw hammer
2. adjustable wrench
3. Vise-Grips
4. combination pliers/cutters
5. bevel-edged chisels, set of three common sizes
6. multi tool
7. retractable, locking tape measure
8. mini level
9. screwdrivers, set of three flathead and three Phillips head or crosshead
10. handsaw, for coarse wood cuts
11. small hacksaw, with extra blades for fine cuts
12. cordless drill, with a kit including metal, masonry, wood, and auger bits, hole cutters, nut drivers, and screwdriver heads

In addition, the Hahns had a stepladder, a workbench, a hand truck, and the average bucket full of miscellaneous material that had accumulated over the years that could be put to use for this kind of project: extension cord, scrapers, utility knife, calculator, work gloves, an awl, a nail set, a two-quart bottle full of various nails and screws, a stud finder, an electrical screwdriver tester, electrical tape, Teflon plumbing tape, dust masks, safety goggles. They also had various wood scraps from old projects and some basic gardening tools.

In my first consultation with the Hahns, I showed them how to access DIY instructions for almost any project on the Internet and then advised them to arm themselves with a comprehensive do-it-yourself home improvement book so they would still have that information when the computers fail. These books tell the owner how his or her home is constructed and how it functions. They offer the essential information on tools, materials, and safety, and they provide step-by-step instructions for repairs or remodeling. They also give advice on choosing outside help and lay out the basics of common building practices. Dale and Crystal were able to find a five-hundred-page manual for ten dollars in the budget section at a local Borders.

In order to break up the costs and define the steps, Dale and Crystal divided the task into three priorities: Food/Water Sustainability, Home Security, and Power/Energy. They then listed specific vulnerabilities, and for each one they listed what actions they could reasonably afford to take to mitigate it, keeping in mind the $2,000 limit, and divided those action items as equally as possible over the next twelve months:

	FOCUS	STEPS
1	Food/Water Sustainability – Garden Total expenses: $69	1. 2 32-gallon garbage can composters - $32 2. Elevated garden bed, 2 x 6 x 8 - $12 (lumber) 3. Self-watering 5-gallon planter - $7 (buckets) 4. Kiddie pool planter (old, from storage) - $0 5. Book: *The Urban Homesteader* - $18
2	Home Security – Doors & Alarms Total expenses: $179	1. Solid-core door, main entrance - $55 DIY 2. Keyed knob/dead bolt lock combo - $56 DIY 3. Doorjamb reinforcement – supplies on hand - $0 4. Peephole - $8 5. Dog – adoption fees, shots, license - $60

	FOCUS	STEPS
3	Energy/ Power Total expenses: $193	1. 1,000-watt gas-powered generator - $150 2. Book: *Living off the Grid* - $13 3. 25-foot multioutlet extension cord - $30
4	Food/Water Sustainabil- ity Total expenses: $158	1. Book: *What to Do When the Shit Hits the Fan* - $13 2. Water storage: at least .5 gallon per person per expected day. Use any old clean beverage containers. - $0 3. Water harvesting: soaker-hose garbage can - $25 for can, hose, fixtures 4. Food storage: canned & dried staples - $90 5. Dog food storage: dry and canned - $30
5	Home Security – Windows & Walls, Gates & Garage Total expenses: $138	1. 0.009-inch security window laminate, 64 square feet - $126, including installation kit 2. Window locks - $9, including stopper dowels 3. Courtyard gate latch, reinforce-ment - $3 for the bolt 4. Garage door, reinforcement via stand-by deadman weights – $0, from materials on hand 5. Curtains for all windows, already installed - $0

	FOCUS	STEPS
6	Energy – Solar Total expenses: $217 Total to date: $954	1. 55-watt Coleman solar kit with controller and 200-watt inverter - $217
7	Food/Water Sustainability – Cooking & Fuel Storage ⁞ Total expenses: $261	1. Generator fuel, to run for one hour every day for 90 days, including fuel (20 gallons), stabilizer, and 4 5-gallon storage cans - $135 2. Propane (BBQ) grill, already owned - $0 3. Camping-style propane heater, already owned - $0 4. Propane fuel, three new, full 20-gallon tanks. These are in addition to the one already hooked to the grill. Each tank fuels slightly under 434,000 BTUs. The Hahns elected to store enough fuel to run their heater and one burner of the grill at medium heat (9,000 for the heater, 5,500 for the burner) for one hour per day for 90 days. - $126
8	Food/Water Sustainability – Farming Total expenses: $180	1. Selection of seeds & seedlings - $180

	FOCUS	STEPS
9	Energy – Hybrid System Total expenses: $249	1. Battery bank: 2 sealed lead acid 12-volt x 115 AH (amp-hour) deep-cycle batteries - $150. More should be added later when funds are available, to increase the bank capacity. 2. 1,100-watt inverter - $89 Note: Inverters are rated for peak or surge power (the power needed to start the contraption) and continuous or running power. Peak power requirements are often 50 to 100 percent more than running power requirements, especially on appliances that contain electric motors. The Hahns' inverter has a 2,200-watt peak power, and can handle either their small refrigerator or their 750-watt microwave. For a discussion on how to find the wattage of an appliance, refer to *Living off the Grid.*
10	Home Security – Lighting & Surveillance	1. 2 wired cameras - $82 2. Radio Shack AV switch - $16 3. TV and other materials on hand - $0 4. Motion-sensing lighting (rigged to run on battery or backup power systems) for courtyard, rear patio, driveway - $68.

	FOCUS	STEPS
	Total expenses: $264	The Hahns chose 4 battery-operated LED motion-detector spots. These lamps last nearly a year on 3 D cells, giving the equivalent of a 20-watt halogen lamp. This allows them an extra lamp without the hassle of keeping the mini solar chargers functioning, and at a significant savings. 5. 15 D cell rechargeable batteries and 2 6 bay universal battery chargers (to be run on the inverter or generator) - $98
11	Home Security – Defense Total expenses: $223	1. 12-guage shotgun - $177 with trigger lock. 2. 50 rounds 12-gauge 00 buckshot - $46
12	Medical and Communications Total expenses: $135	1. Prepacked group-sized first aid kit. The Hahns chose a comprehensive "base camp" kit at Target - $35. 2. Common OTC meds already on hand. $0 Note: This should include a generous supply of diphenhydramine HCl for minor allergic reactions and sleep. 3. One single adult course each of meds recommended, prescribed, and explained thoroughly by the family doctor (your doctor may prescribe something else):

FOCUS	STEPS
Total expense, entire project: $1985	a. Cephalexin 500 mg tablets for skin, ear, urinary, and upper respiratory infections b. Azithromycin 250 mg tablets for respiratory infections c. Albuterol sulfate inhaler for respiratory emergencies (asthma, etc). d. Nitroglycerin 0.4 mg tablets for heart-related chest pain e. Epinephrine auto injector for severe allergic reactions (anaphylaxis) f. Hydrocodone – acetaminophen 5-500 for pain and diarrhea The Hahns co-pay: $30 4. GMRS long-range radios, 2-pack, with charger/rechargeable batteries - $70 5. Online first aid training - free

The Hahns barely squeaked by with these additional expenses, but in the end, they accomplished what they had set out to do. After careful consideration, they decided their retreat budget for the next twelve months would be half of what they spent the first year.

The Hahns began again by listing priorities, such as the following:

1. Expanding the battery bank (increase to six or eight batteries) and an additional 55-watt solar power kit.

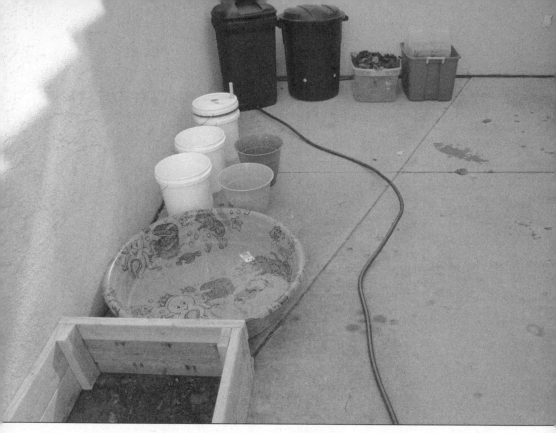

The Hahns new urban farm. A raised bed, some buckets and pots, a kiddie pool, water collector with gravity-powered soaker hose, and compositor.

2. Buying a more powerful inverter.
3. Purchasing a 9mm pistol and boosting the supply of ammo.
4. Taking a Wilderness first aid course and expanding the medical kit.
5. Storing additional food, water, and fuel.
6. Getting professional firearms training.

COMMUNITY - The Rockville Ranch (name changed and location suppressed to protect the residents).

The Rockville Ranch is located in the high desert of the Southwest, thirty miles from the closest small town and a hundred miles from the nearest city. It is accessed by a ten-mile stretch of dirt road from the highway to the east, and from that approach, it is completely hidden from view by the five-hundred-foot high sandstone mountain that encompasses it.

Approximately forty homes and community structures are blasted into the rock or built along its base. At any time, the community will house between eighty and two hundred residents.

Among the structures blasted into the rock are a large twelve-apartment complex, a chapel, a restaurant, a community "conversation pit" and a meeting center.

Tunnels punching through the mountain from south to north provide travel and escape routes, and at least one of the residences has entrances on both sides of the mountain. A ladder system provides access to the top of the mountain where the desert for miles around can be observed without difficulty. The continuing construction implies the presence of high explosives, and the large firing range leaves little doubt the community is suitably armed.

Rockville has extensive food storage supplemented by large crop fields, orchards, a chicken farm, cattle, and a dairy. Water is provided by wells, and the potential for water harvesting is excellent due to the configuration of the mountain, nearby streambeds, and large potholes on the sandstone.

There are many private passenger vehicles as well as heavy utility and construction vehicles and machinery. Although most of the vehicles rely on gasoline provided by a community gravity fuel pump, the bulk of the community's energy and power needs are supplied by extensive solar arrays and wind turbines backed up by diesel-powered generators. Cell service from towers on a nearby mountain range and satellite dishes give access to modern communications technologies.

Although the residents take advantage of available services in two larger towns about forty miles to the southeast and northeast, the Rockville Ranch seems entirely self-sustainable, even down to its own social and community services. Schooling is done at home and there's a community day care.

The Rockville Ranch got its start back in the mid-1970s when the founder, an excommunicated Mormon polygamist with a bigamy conviction, sought "another Ark"; a haven where his friends and family would be safe from the chaos of the world and the impending apocalypse. But there's at least one problem: it is leased land. Some of the residents are nervous about the fact that the BLM lease is up in fifteen years.

The Rockville community is friendly and doesn't feel the need to hide what they're doing or how sustainable they are. Indeed, Rockville Ranch presents a formidable defensive position against intruders from the ground or the air. Unlike Waco or Ruby Ridge, a small federal incursion here would be very unlikely and could easily be repulsed. This is perhaps why the state appears to ignore the ranch and why Rockville stands out as an example of a successful retreat.

GOVERNMENT

CMOC, the Cheyenne Mountain Operations Center, is housed two thousand feet into Cheyenne Mountain just outside of Colorado Springs and Fort Carson, Colorado. It's built to withstand a

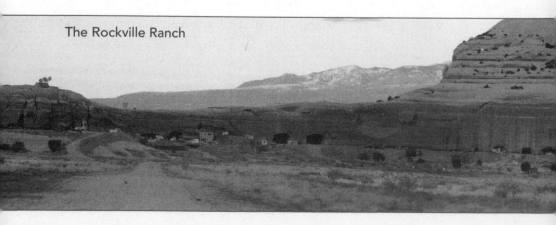

The Rockville Ranch

thirty-megaton blast within one nautical mile and has metal walls and a long tunnel to mitigate the effects of an EMP.

Other U.S. COG (continuity of government) shelters built by DOD or FEMA included the following:

- Project Greek Island, located beneath the Greenbriar Hotel in Virginia. This shelter was built in 1960 and was decommissioned in 1992.
- Raven Rock Mountain Complex was a facility built in the '50s in Pennsylvania.
- The Mount Weather civilian command center is a FEMA facility in Virginia.

Certainly, shelters to protect large numbers of military officials and politicians are no surprise, but what about sheltering the masses? In Switzerland, two interesting shelters were built by the government. The first was the Redoubt Fortress system. The second was the Sonnenberg Tunnel. This was a motorway tunnel built in 1976 with the world's largest civilian fallout shelter, essentially an underground metropolis complete with a command center, a complex air-filtration system, a prison, and a hospital with beds for up to 350 patients. It was originally said to have a

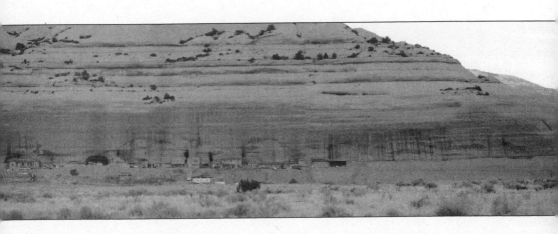

twenty-thousand-person capacity, but after a 1987 practice drill proved that it would take two weeks for it to actually become operational (it took two days just to close the five-foot- thick exterior doors), the capacity was downgraded to two thousand. With the reality that these kinds of shelters would become management nightmares, Switzerland once again relied on shelters in cellars of houses and apartment blocks. A law passed during the 1960s requires space for every resident in a nuclear shelter, thus there are over a quarter of a million of them. Public shelters can be under schools, fire departments, sports stadiums, or in parking garages. Many families have private shelters in their homes. In fact, according to a widely ignored law, every Swiss household is required to have and stock its own shelter. And, to complete the "retreat" image, every household is required to maintain a firearm.

Chapter 8

The Prepared Traveler – Establishing a Personal Retreat Zone

As an international traveler whose purposes for being in third world countries were sometimes suspect, I have often found myself under direct attack by antagonist groups. This has included a cell phone bomb planted at my Georgian hotel, dynamiting of my Bolivian pension, threats by angry armed Arab tribesmen, strafing by aircraft, standoffs with unhappy rebel soldiers, mob attacks, and simple robberies and assaults. I have spent many nights doing what little can be done to turn my temporary quarters into a functioning retreat.

It's these experiences that have prompted this chapter. We are a nation of travelers, and a good percentage of us will be nowhere near our planned retreats when whatever evil is going to happen happens. As the world gets smaller and smaller, it's far more likely that the average person will need a real retreat from occasional threats of isolated criminal or terrorist violence than from any zombie attack or doomsday scenario.

It stands to reason that one can't predict when things are going to go to hell in a handbasket. There are no safe rooms in cheap hotels, no panic rooms in restaurants, no retreats in the client's office, no bomb shelters in taxis. What follows here are some methods of improvising what we'll call a "personal retreat zone" when you're traveling.

1. Make certain somebody you absolutely trust knows your travel plans in detail.
2. Consider a concealed weapon. This requires planning ahead. In the United States, you must have a permit. Firearms are illegal in many countries. In others, automatic weapons and explosives can be purchased by anyone at the local market. If you can't get a firearm and ammunition in your target country, a Taser or pepper spray is a weaker but reasonable substitute.
3. Consider carrying a burglar bar in your luggage. This device fits under any doorknob (they're telescoping and adjustable). One end has a hard rubber floor pad that locks onto wood, tile, carpet, or cement. For emergencies, just kick the bottom of the brace away from the floor. A cheap but less effective alternative is a simple rubber or wood wedge doorstop.
4. Consider putting together a travel security kit consisting of several door/window screamer contacts and a motion detector or two, a couple of window track locks or a telescoping "Charlie Bar," a roll of heavy-duty tape, and a door wedge. With the exception of a Charlie Bar or burglar bar, the whole kit can fit into a small backpack. The kit should also include a very minimal seventy-two-hour supply of food and hydration. You will be fine locked in a hotel room for a few days with two liters of water and a handful of high-calorie energy bars or an MRE.
5. Avoid taking a room on the first floor. Before choosing a room, remember higher floors are more secure from intruders, but the lower floors are easier to escape or be rescued from. Choose your poison.

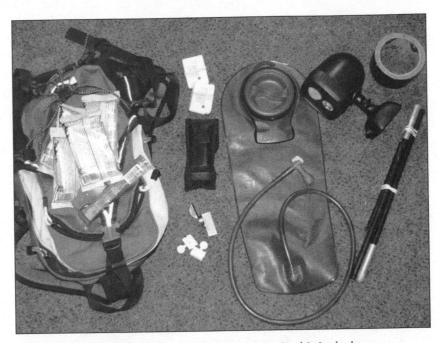

My personal third world travel retreat security kit includes a sectional dowel (made from an old tent frame rod), a multitool, two nails (to pin the hinge on outward-opening doors), strong tape, two door/window screamers, three window/sliding door track locks, a motion-detecting spot lamp (to be aimed directly at the entrance door to blind intruders), a 72-hour supply of water and calories, and some cash. A burglar bar or a simple door wedge is often added, and on occasion a weapon of some kind is included.

6. Choose a room that is close but not next to elevators and stairways. If someone you don't know is exiting from an elevator on your floor, let them out first and then go to another floor or the lobby if they act suspicious.

7. Once you get the lay of the building and surroundings, preplan an escape route and a contingency.

8. Be one with your inner *MacGyver* and *Burn Notice* fantasies, but remember: about 99 percent of that doesn't actually work as it does on TV.

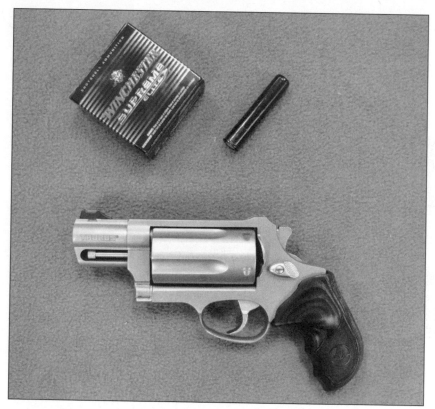

The perfect traveling companion? The Public Defender variant of the Taurus handgun, "The Judge," is a five-shot revolver that shoots a .45 caliber round or a .410 shot shell. It's small and light, built and promoted as a concealable self-defense or home protection weapon. The photo shows the handgun and a box of Winchester Supreme Elite .410 shells. The shells contain twelve plated BBs and three plated cylinder projectiles, providing stopping power and protection from overpenetration. Loading a Public Defender with alternating .45 and WSE .410 rounds results in a formidable close-quarters personal defense weapon.

9. Watch diligently for suspicious people on the premises. Don't trust anybody. Intruders will pretend to be someone else (hotel security, room service, pizza man, etc.).

10. Make sure the hotel/motel or apartment and surrounding grounds look secure before paying for the room. Do not take

a room with large windows above the head of the bed that open into an interior courtyard. Avoid rooms with balconies.

11. Beware of rooms that have adjoining rooms. Be sure an adjoining room is locked with a secure deadbolt.

12. The room entrance should have a solid-core hardwood or metal door with deadbolts that have a throw of at least one

Good door security in an inexpensive stateside motel room. The features of this self-closing, self-locking door are a solid hardwood core, an upper and lower peephole, a card-activated dead bolt with a one-inch-plus throw, a swing bar lock, and a wood door wedge.

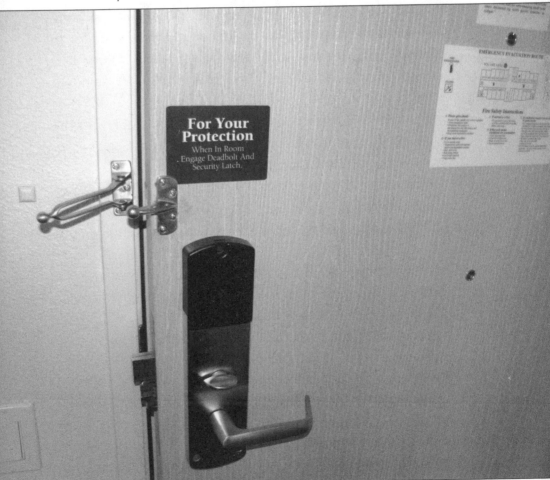

inch and push-button knob locks. If possible, the door should be self-closing and self-locking, and electronic card access is a plus. The door should also have a wide-angle peephole.

13. Use the dead bolt and any other locks on the door. If you're really paranoid, take twenty minutes to pin the hinges if they're on the outside of the entrance door. Bathroom doors typically open out, with the hinges on the outside. Pinning the bathroom door may give you the few minutes you need to get out a bathroom window … just make sure there's a window if that's your plan. Pinning is easy to do with a multitool and a couple of nails.

14. Use the peephole before answering the door. From inside the room, demand to see an ID, even if the visitors are in uniform. Have them slip it under the door so you can see it clearly, then call the front desk to verify the reason they are standing outside your door.

15. Once you've cleared the intruders, open the door with the chain lock or swing bar engaged to conduct business, but do not rely on a chain lock to stop an intruder.

16. Do not leave windows open. Close them and lock them or place a dowel in the frame track or apply clamp locks that only allow the window to open a few inches for ventilation. If you have screamer contacts, apply them to the entrance door and windows with a loop of strong tape. Do not use the double-sided tape that comes in the contact screamer package as it's extremely difficult to remove.

17. Worrisome windows can be reinforced with strong tape. In the United States, most high-end hotels are glazed with safety or security glass. Not so in other countries or in very low-end hotels stateside. Tape provides a surprisingly effective barrier against penetration of shattered glass, similar to that of the clear security laminates mentioned earlier. Probably the most effective tape for this purpose is Hurricane Tape. Check out

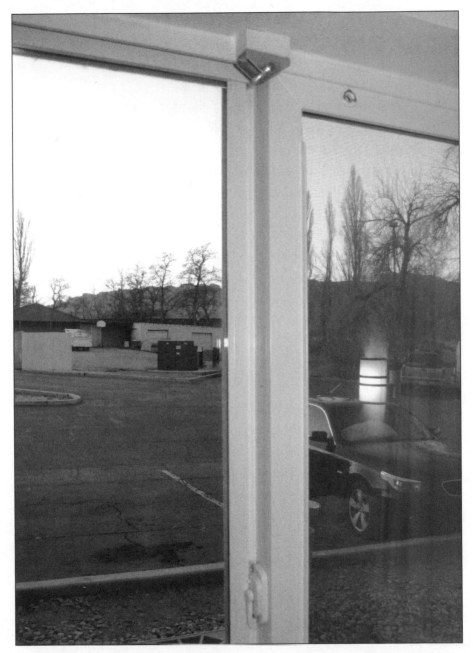

Good window security in the same ground-floor room: double panes of security glass, a fastener to lock the sliding window to the frame, and a bolt or pin that can be set to lock the window closed or open slightly for ventilation.

this website for a better description and videos of product tests:

web.archive.org/web/20130725115219/http://bunkerinc
.com/hurricane.htm

Unfortunately, Hurricane Tape is hard to come by unless you live along the East Coast. Contrary to what we're told on disaster websites, heavy-duty duct tape performed acceptably in my own impact and ballistic tests. Heavy-duty woven or thick clear plastic packing tape performed almost identically well, and these tapes are far easier to find stateside and overseas.

The decision to tape means leaving a mess behind on the window. If you decide to tape, tape over the entire window, ovelapping strips in two layers, one horizontal and one vertical. Double-back the end of each strip so it provides a tab that will make removal easier.

18. Do not leave sliding glass balcony doors open, even on upper floors.
19. Keep the curtains closed.
20. If you're worried about seriously violent intruders, do not sleep where anyone would assume you would. For example, pull the mattress off the bed and move it to the bathroom or take a mini bedroll to throw wherever you'd like, then fluff the real bed so it looks like somebody is asleep there.
21. If you're going out ...
    a. keep the room very neat so it will be easy to notice anything disturbed as you enter the room,
    b. make a habit of leaving a light on. If you return and it's off, you'll know something's wrong.
22. In restaurants and other public places, learn to go into PRZ-mode automatically:
    a. Sit near other people or near aisles or doors.

b. Sit with your back toward a nearby wall looking outward toward the entrance and occupants.
c. Quickly preplan an escape route and contingency.
d. Stay sober.
e. Do not discuss plans or family in an open area or with strangers.

A company called *onPoint Tactical* offers a course called *Urban Escape and Evasion*. Reviews of this course have been very good. The only complaint is that it's expensive (around $800 for three days), but like other good things, you get what you pay for. The intensive curriculum is urban survival from the James Bond-ish perspective (lock picking, vehicle pursuit, escape from restraints, etc.), and nearly everyone who takes it swears it's the most fun they've ever had. The website:

onpointtactical.com/services/urban-escape-and-evasion

CHAPTER 9

Retreats in the Media

THESE SOURCES HAVE SOME RELEVANCE TO SURVIVALIST RETREATS, though admittedly in some cases not much.

MOVIES

The Beach (2000) – A wandering American gets more than he can handle in a secret Thai island community.

The Book of Eli (2010) – A man travels on a mission to protect a sacred book that contains the secrets to mankind's survival.

The Crazies (2010) – A small Iowa town is ravaged by zombie-ish insane people after an accidental release of toxins into the water supply.

Dawn of the Dead (1978 and 2004) – Survivors of a zombie plague take refuge. Both versions are classics.

Day of the Triffids (1964 movie; 2009 TV miniseries) – Celestial disturbances blind 99 percent of the population, and an invasion by alien plants ensues.

Defiance (2008) – Brothers flee into the Belarusian forests where they join Russian resistance fighters and build a retreat to protect a large refugee Jewish group.

Deliverance (1972) – A group of friends get an unpleasant reception when they take a river trip into Deep South backcountry.

I Am Legend (2008) – One of a few survivors of a zombie plague tries valiantly to find a cure. It's a classic adaptation of

Matheson's novel of the same name, one of many adaptations since *The Last Man on Earth* (1964). Vincent Price plays a sole survivor of a living-dead plague.

Mad Max 2 (Road Warrior) (1981) – In post-apocalypse Australia Mel Gibson saves a retreat community from the marauding hordes.

Mad Max Beyond Thunderdome (1985) – Mel Gibson works two—yes, two—retreats: a sleazebag tech town and a colony of children.

Malevil (1972) – Buddies are in a castle wine cellar and survive nuclear armageddon. They attempt to rebuild a society which must be protected from the evil surviving neighbors.

No Blade of Grass (1970) – A family heads to Scotland when a virus devastates London.

Omega Man (1971) – A self-immunized scientist in L.A. survives germ warfare only to be forced to deal with vampirish zombie hordes of pissed-off survivors. This was an early adaptation of the *I Am Legend* theme.

Packin' It In (1983) – A comedy in which families flee to the mountains from strange afflictions in L.A.

Panic in the Year Zero (1962) – Before *Red Dawn*, this was the ultimate survivalist movie. It's still one of the best and most believable. Nuclear bombs destroy L.A. and other large cities around the world while a family is on a camping trip, and Dad fights to save the family while local society goes to hell in a handbasket.

The Postman (1997) – A con man finds his life's calling delivering mail to post-apocalypse survivors.

Ravenous (1999) – Soldiers, cannibalism, and Indian demon legends combine in a rather gruesome story set near the Sierra Nevada mountains in the mid-19th century.

Red Dawn (1984 and 2011) – This is *the* classic survivalist movie in which all-American high school kids fight communist invaders, Russians/Cubans in 1984 and North Koreans in 2011.

Reign of Fire (2002) – Years after a plague of fire-breathing dragons take over, a team of dragon-slayer specialists join a local survivor community to destroy the dragons and regain control.

The Road (2009) – Vigo plays the role of a man who will do anything to keep his son alive in a post-apocalypse mess.

The Stand (1994 TV miniseries) – A plague decimates the planet and confused survivors of a small town must deal with the forces of good and evil waging war among them.

The Survivors (1983) - Two strangers end up in a survival retreat preparing for battle after a joint encounter with a hit man who pursues them.

Swiss Family Robinson (1960) – A family is shipwrecked on a deserted island and prepares to do battle with pirates.

Tank Girl (1995) – After a comet wastes, the earth and water becomes scarce, Tank girl does battle against water-monopolizing giant corporations.

Terminator: Judgment Day (1991) – Bad-cyborg-turned-hero Arnold schwarzenegger strives to protect Sarah Connor and her son from an advanced cyborg from hell. This movie contains only a very few references regarding retreats but for some unknown reason is often cited by survivalists as a classic retreat movie.

Tremors (1990) – A group of survivors in a small town do battle against the giant wormlike underground creatures that have surrounded their town and killed off their neighbors. Reba McEntire and Michael Gross are hysterically funny in their roles as classic survivalists.

Twelve Monkeys (1995) – In a disease-devastated future, Bruce Willis is sent back in time to find out what happened.

Waterworld (1995) – Global warming has melted the ice caps and flooded the earth. Costner plays a mutant human with gills and webbed digits who fights off the marauding marine hordes and helps a woman and a child find dry land.

2012 (2009) – A global disaster destroys the world. The chosen few are to be saved on specially prepared "arks" while the have-nots are left to their own resources.

FICTION PRINT

Alas, Babylon, Pat Frank, 1959 – An excellent book by author Frank (Hart) written as he watched the Cold War unfold. The plot involves a nuclear holocaust predicted by the hero, who stockpiles provisions. Disorder prevails but eventually, human spirit and love triumph. Spark notes at: www.sparknotes.com/lit/alas/context.html

The Day of the Triffids, John Wyndham, 1951 – see the movie summary.

Deliverance, 1970 – see the movie summary.

Dies the Fire, 2004, S. M. Stirling – This is the first in the Emberverse series by Stirling. "The Change" alters science and technology, resulting in the demise of society and infrastructure. The protagonist battles evil survivalists, rotten lawmen, cannibals, etc.

Earth Abides, George Stewart, 1949 – Civilization is obliterated by disease and survivors adapt.

Ecotopia, Ernest Callenbach, 1975 – This book appeals to left-leaning hippie-style idealists. The story is about Ecotopia, a new country formed by the succession of several western U.S. states to escape the evils of materialism. Listen closely and you can hear the kumbayahs.

Ecotopia Emerging, Ernest Callenbach, 1981 – More of the same.

Farnham's Freehold, Robert Heinlein, 1964 – Farnham's retreat backfires and sends him into a new universe where his family is doomed to slavery.

Lucifer's Hammer, Pournelle and Niven, 1977 – Another comet story. This comet causes all sorts of secondary natural disasters that destroy civilization and bring on a new ice age. Appropriate struggles ensue.

Malevil, Robert Merle, 1972 – See the movie description.

Patriots: A Novel of Survival in the Coming Collapse, James Wesley Rawles, 2009 – During global economic pandemonium, a Chicago group of survivalists escape to their Idaho retreat. This book first appeared in the late 90s but was republished in 2009. Considering the recent economic pandemonium it's not surprising the republished book was a best seller.

The Postman, David Brin, 1985 – See the movie description.

The Road, Cormac McCarthy, 2006 – See the movie description.

The Stand, Stephen King, 1978 – See the movie description.

Tomorrow!, Phillip Wylie, 1954 – This is the story of families in two neighboring Midwest cities dealing with an atomic bomb attack. Wylie is by far the most interesting and prolific of the early sci-fi survivalism writers.

Tunnel in the Sky, Robert Heinlein, 1955 – A survival class somehow finds itself stranded at the end of a cosmic tunnel. The students must work together cooperatively to stay alive.

Wolf and Iron, Gordon R. Dickinson, 1993 – Financial collapse destroys civilization. The hero must cross a plundered, hostile countryside to find safe haven at a Montana ranch.

World Made by Hand, James Howard Kunstler, 2008 – Horrific terrorism, economic collapse, and a pandemic decimate the population and force the government to flee. Cutoff survivors try to rebuild their lives in a dark, violent, dangerous new world.

NONFICTION PRINT

Barnyard in Your Backyard: A Beginner's Guide to Raising Chickens, Ducks, Geese, Rabbits, Goats, Sheep, and Cattle, Gail Damerow, 2002

Dancing at Armageddon: Survivalism and Chaos in Modern Times, Richard G. Mitchell Jr., 2001 – This is an exceptional, insightful look at survivalists and survivalism by a participant-observer sociologist.

Fallout Protection, 1961 – A government booklet released in 1961. See it as a pdf here: www.orau.org/ptp/Library/cdv/h-6.pdf

FM 5-15 Field Fortifications, U.S. Army, 1944 – See it as a pdf here: www.ibiblio.org/hyperwar/USA/ref/FM/PDFs/FM5-15.44.pdf

How to Survive the H-Bomb and Why, Pat Frank, 1962 – A classic how-to from the writer of the novel *Alas, Babylon*.

Home Power Magazine – Not a survivalist magazine or site but a fantastic newsstand or online resource for information on sustainable living and small-scale renewable energy. www.homepower.com/home-efficiency

Living off the Grid, David Black, 2008

The Long Emergency, James H. Kunstler, 2005 – Non-fiction predictions and advice from the author of *World Made by Hand*.

Mother Earth News – A country-style and sustainable-living magazine with subtle undertones of survivalism. Very informative.

Nuclear War Survival Skills, Cresson Kearny, 1979 and 1992 – At the time of this writing, this is available as a free download at this website: oism.org/nwss/nwss.pdf

Survival Under Atomic Attack, 1950 – Another government booklet, downloadable here: www.orau.org/ptp/Library/cdv/Survival%20Under%20Atomic%20Attack.pdf

Tappan on Survival, Mel Tappan, 1981 – This is one of the classics written by an early leader of the survivalist movement.

When All Hell Breaks Loose, Cody Lundin, 2007

What to Do When the Shit Hits the Fan, David Black, 2006

Television

There are a myriad of TV movies and series (e.g., *24, Six Feet Under, Lost, Terminator: The Sarah Connors Chronicles,* etc.) that have a minor character or subplot that could be survivalist-related. They're often touted as survivalist media references but in actuality, many have little to do with the realities of survivalism or survival retreats. Here are a few exceptions:

The Colony – A Discovery reality series that follows groups attempting to survive under simulated conditions of a global catastrophe.

The Day After – A 1983 TV movie about events before and after a three-hundred-plus Soviet ICBM nuclear attack on the United States.

Jericho – A 2006 series following the story of Jericho, Kansas, in the wake of a massive nuclear attack on the United States.

The Fire Next Time – A 1993 miniseries about the struggle of a family to survive the catastrophic effects of global warming and the resulting chaos.

Survivor – A competitive "reality" series in which contestants are shown surviving in remote, austere conditions. Thought of by this author as embarrassingly lame and unrealistic, it seems to focus on egos and testosterone more than realistic survival scenarios but does give some interesting glimpses into survival psychology.

Survivors – A 1975–77 and 2008 BBC series about a group that survives a horrible plague.

Threads – A grim 1984 BBC TV movie about a couple of families and politicians in Sheffield as they deal with nuclear war.

WEBSITES, BLOGS, FORUMS

americanpreppersnetwork.com
survivalblog.com
textfiles.com/survival

VIDEO GAMES

Fallout (1997) – This video game classic uses a protagonist who has survived nuclear holocaust in the government shelters (the Vaults) and is forced to leave the safety of the vault to find a replacement chip vital to its water recycler. *Fallout 2*, *Fallout 3*, and *Fallout 4* are now available.

MUSIC

"Year Zero", Nine Inch Nails (2007) – An interesting album with references to a future dystopia that resulted from events and policies of the present.